Weight Training for the Young Athlete

Weight Training
FOR

NEW YORK   1980   ATHENEUM

Dr. Frederick C. Hatfield

THE
Young Athlete

Library of Congress Cataloging in Publication Data

Hatfield, Frederick C.
  Weight training for the young athlete.

  1. Weight lifting.   2. Physical fitness.
3. Sports—Training.   I. Title.
GV546.H38   1980   796.4'1   79-55614
ISBN 0-689-11041-3

Copyright © 1980 by Frederick C. Hatfield
All rights reserved
Published simultaneously in Canada by
  McClelland and Stewart Ltd.
Composition by Connecticut Printers, Inc.,
  Bloomfield, Connecticut
Printed and bound by Halliday Lithograph Corporation,
  Hanover, Massachusetts
Designed by Kathleen Carey
First Edition

ACKNOWLEDGMENTS

Photographs of exercises:
  BLOND BOY: Freddy Hatfield
  DARK-HAIRED BOY: Steve Churchwell
  GIRL: Laurel Mills

The author would like to thank Laurel, Steve, and Freddy for their kind assistance in preparing this book for young athletes—also, the neighborhood kids for reading the book and offering their expert comments on how a book should be written for children of their ages. Freddy, the author's son, has been training with his dad for some time and was especially helpful in the preparation of this book and in the decision to write it in the first place. Thanks also to the Madison Weightlifting Center and the Continental Spa of Madison for the use of their facilities.

Contents

PREFACE   ix

A NOTE TO PARENTS AND COACHES   3

1: WHAT IS AN ATHLETE?   10

     AN ATHLETE IS STRONG   11

     AN ATHLETE HAS ENDURANCE   12

     AN ATHLETE IS FAST   13

     AN ATHLETE IS AGILE   13

     AN ATHLETE HAS GOOD BALANCE   14

     AN ATHLETE IS FLEXIBLE   15

     AN ATHLETE IS COORDINATED   16

2: HOW TO BECOME AN ATHLETE   18

     FIRST YOU MUST BE PHYSICALLY FIT   18

     PART OF BEING FIT IS EATING GOOD FOOD   20

     YOU MUST LISTEN TO YOUR COACH   22

3: LIFTING WEIGHTS FOR PHYSICAL FITNESS   25

     HOW TO LIFT WEIGHTS FOR

         EACH PART OF FITNESS   25

     HOW TO DO EACH EXERCISE   29

     EXERCISES FOR THE ARMS   31

     EXERCISES FOR THE SHOULDERS   34

     EXERCISES FOR THE UPPER BACK AND SPINE   40

     EXERCISES FOR THE CHEST   45

     EXERCISES FOR THE HIPS AND UPPER LEGS   47

     EXERCISES FOR THE LOWER LEGS   52

4: SOME HINTS FOR YOUNG ATHLETES ON TRAINING FOR FITNESS   53

     SOME EXERCISES THAT SHOULD

         ALWAYS BE DONE   53

EXERCISES THAT SHOULD NOT BE DONE   54

SEE YOUR DOCTOR FOR A CHECKUP OFTEN   55

KEEPING RECORDS OF YOUR PROGRESS   56

BOYS AND GIRLS BOTH BENEFIT FROM
    LIFTING WEIGHTS   57

HOW TO GET STARTED IN WEIGHT TRAINING
    FOR FITNESS   58

**5: GUIDELINES FOR
SPORT CONDITIONING**   60

SOME IMPORTANT THINGS TO REMEMBER   61

SOME BASIC RULES FOR CONDITIONING
    IN ALL SPORTS   65

OFF-SEASON TRAINING   67

PRE-SEASON TRAINING   68

IN-SEASON TRAINING   68

**6: WEIGHT-TRAINING AND
CONDITIONING PROGRAMS FOR SPORTS**   71

FOOTBALL   72

GYMNASTICS   78

WRESTLING   81

SWIMMING   84

BASKETBALL   89

OTHER SPORTS   92

Glossary   95

Appendix One: SOME CALISTHENTICS THAT
CAN BE DONE WHEN WEIGHTS ARE NOT
AVAILABLE —OR FOR WARMING UP   103

Appendix Two: SOME STRETCHING EXERCISES
TO BE DONE FOR FLEXIBILITY BEFORE
AND AFTER WORKOUTS   109

Appendix Three: AN EXAMPLE OF AN
ATHLETE'S TRAINING RECORD   116

Preface

Many grown-ups believe that lifting weights is dangerous for children. "Lifting weights will stunt your growth," they say. Or, "You could hurt yourself." Some grown-ups even believe that "girls should be girls, and play only girl games, and leave sports to the boys." If these grown-ups only knew what the great coaches and some doctors know about sports and exercise, they would never say such things, for they are not true.

Training with dumbbells and barbells can actually make you much healthier, more physically fit, and a better athlete. The problem is that very few people know enough about how children should exercise. This is the purpose of this book. It will teach you how to become healthier, more physically fit, and a better athlete by training with dumbbells and barbells in the proper way.

This book is meant for both boys and girls between the ages of eight and twelve years old. Older children can benefit from the book, also. But it is important to show the book to your parents and your gym teachers, especially, for they can help you in finding a good place to lift weights, and one where you can get plenty of help in doing your exercises correctly and safely.

Enjoy your exercises. But above all, remember to do the exercises properly and in a safe manner.

Dr. Frederick C. Hatfield
University of Wisconsin/Madison

Weight Training for
the Young Athlete

A Note to Parents and Coaches

CHILDREN CAN benefit from prudent weight training. Properly applied stress, in the form of resistive-type exercises, such as calisthenics and weight-training techniques, can do much for:

1. *Improving tonus in skeletal muscles.* Children's muscles have grown faster than the attendant skeletal structure, making movements somewhat jerky and uncoordinated on account of the looseness.

2. *Improving skill.* By tightening these loose muscles, movements are somewhat smoother, since the "slack" is taken up between the muscle and skeleton. This allows the child to experience more accurate movement patterns, and therefore acquire skills more quickly.

3

3. *Reducing sport-related injuries.* Stronger muscles hold joints together better than weak muscles. Also, greater skill in various movements tends to diminish the possibilities of injury as well.

4. *Preparing the youngster for sports later on.* By concentrating on improving the various components of physical fitness at an early age, the youngster will be many steps ahead in mastering competitive-sport techniques later in his or her childhood years.

5. *Improving the child's self-confidence.* Owing to the greater strength acquired through weight training, as well as the general improvement in all areas of physical fitness, the child will naturally become more self-assured when setting out to master a new movement or skill. Also, training allows the child to become keenly aware of his or her physical limitations.

Unfortunately, many myths and old wives' tales have persisted in the general field of weight lifting, which have served to make coaches and parents skeptical about allowing their children to lift weights. Often these misconceptions arose because of improperly applied weight-training procedures. The fact is that:

1. *Weight training does not stunt a child's growth.* There is no evidence that weight training causes bones to harden any faster than normal. The fact that, in the past, the great strong men were generally short was a matter of natural selection—a short

man's more efficient leverage made him better at lifting heavy weights than tall men—and has nothing to do with what weights did to his bones.

2. *Lifting weights can hurt a young child.* This is as true for children as much, or more so, as it is for older people. However, what is advocated in this book is lifting *moderate* weights—*not* very heavy weights. This is a basic principle that old and young alike should adhere to. Also, selection of the proper exercises will do much in curtailing the possibility of injury to the muscles or joints.

3. *Muscles do not turn to fat after training ends.* Muscle tissue and fat tissue are entirely different—one cannot become the other. Sensible weight training will help keep fat from forming, and upon ceasing weight training, the muscles may lose tone or size but will not turn to fat. Generally, fat may form because the athlete's diet was not changed in relation to the decreased activity level. Thus, upon stopping one's training, one should also alter his or her calorie intake.

4. *Girls do not become muscle-bound from lifting weights.* Girls and boys in the age range of eight to twelve are still well in front of the pubertal stage, when their respective hormones begin to be produced, causing signs of maturity to appear. One of the signs for boys is a distinct thickening of the musculature, caused by testosterone, the male hormone. This hormone is only minimally present in girls, making it impossible for them to acquire

the huge musculatures that boys can. For girls as well as boys, proper weight training will not cause muscle-boundness (i.e., loss of flexibility due to unnatural increases in muscle size). Rather, greater flexibility is usually derived because of the even strength and tone acquired in all muscles surrounding each joint.

5. *Huge amounts of weights are not needed to derive benefit.* In fact, children should not lift heavy weights at all—their bones are still soft, and there is a distinct possibility of the muscles' tendons pulling away from the soft bone to which they attach. Also, the heart muscle at this age range is smaller than it should be relative to the size of the rest of the body. Therefore, undue stress upon the heart may cause problems to appear. Weight-training exercises for children should involve weights that the child is capable of lifting easily for about twenty repetitions, although only ten are to be done—in other words, only moderate amounts of weight—not heavy weights—are needed for development of tone, strength, and muscular endurance.

6. *Weight lifting is not bad for the joints.* Strengthening the muscles surrounding each joint actually makes the joint more stable and less susceptible to injury. In fact, mild overload on the ligaments and tendons in the joint region actually serves to thicken them (much the same as callus forming on the hands), making them far stronger than they

6

ordinarily would be. Such a practice must, however, be dealt with cautiously. Extreme stretching of joints can cause damage—only mild stretching with moderate resistance is called for.

These are adults' most common concerns about weight training in general, and about weight training for children in particular. It is hoped that pointing out the reality of each situation will prompt you to give your child guidance and encouragement in his or her training efforts. Training can be fun, especially if the child sees that encouragement is forthcoming from the significant persons in his or her life. Weight training constitutes the single most efficient method known to science for improving strength, power, agility, and tone. Engaged in properly, it can be a very efficient and meaningful tool in helping the child to realize his or her maximal potential in many sport endeavors as well as in the general area of physical fitness.

Following is a list of guidelines to follow in monitoring your child's training. Following these commonsense rules along with the procedures in the child's section of the book will ensure that only good will result from your child's efforts.

1. Lift two or three times weekly, never for more than an hour.
2. Limit each training session to five or six of the most important exercises—more can become boring or perhaps taxing.
3. Do three sets of each exercise, with about ten

repetitions per set, using a weight that can be handled with relative ease.

4. Avoid undue stretching of joints—mild stretching is permissible.

5. Avoid all ballistic-type movements. Control the weight, don't swing it.

6. Avoid movements involving hyperextension of the spine (such as Olympic-style weight-lifting movements, back raises, and deep squatting movements), but definitely engage in exercises that will help strengthen the back muscles. This practice is extremely important, as it will help eliminate back problems later in life.

7. Do sit-ups with knees bent. Never do straight-leg sit-ups, as this places too much stress on the lower spine because of the peculiar arrangement of the muscles involved.

8. In each exercise period spend time on the legs— particularly the muscles in the back of the upper leg—as many knee injuries can be avoided later in life. One common condition that exercising the hamstrings helps to eliminate is called Osgood/ Schlatter's Disease. This debilitating adolescent disease generally results because of uneven pull from thigh and hamstring muscles on the knee joint. By strengthening the hamstrings, the tension is more equalized, thereby minimizing the probability of this condition occurring.

9. Be sure that your child is eating properly. Generally, a child's diet should consist of calories from

fats, carbohydrates, and protein in the following amounts: 20 percent of daily calories from fat sources, 60 percent of daily calories from carbohydrate sources, and 20 percent of daily calories from protein sources. Try to avoid allowing your child to eat junk foods, especially sugar-laden foods. Good eating habits are generally formed in the childhood years, and children often adopt the eating patterns of their parents. Set a good example—your child is important.

10. Don't be afraid to train with your child—you may derive the same fitness benefits yourself! Besides, your child may come to enjoy training more if he or she sees that his or her parents do it too.

11. Should your child have medical problems— particularly but not limited to heart problems, anemia, congenital bone defects, or skeletal/ muscular injuries—consult a reputable sports-medicine specialist. Your family doctor can recommend one.

1: What Is
an Athlete?

So, you want to be an athlete? Have you ever stopped to think about what an athlete is? Is it someone who plays sports? Yes—but, of course, not all people who play sports are athletes. Some people play sports for fun or to become fit, but these people are not athletes. *An athlete becomes fit to play sports.* Think about it. For the athlete, his or her sport is serious business. Not just play or fun, although most athletes do love their sports and enjoy playing them. Athletes are special people who have chosen to excel at their sport, and work very hard to do so. An athlete, together with his or her coach, tries to figure out exactly what kind of fitness the sport they're working for requires. Then he or she follows a systematic conditioning program, so that the athlete is "in shape" to excel at the sport.

Different sports call for different kinds of fitness. A good coach knows this and helps the athlete set up a training program that will help the athlete become good at his or her sport. (For example, a football player's training program has to be different from a gymnast's training program, because these two athletes' sports require different types of fitness. The same is true of soccer players and wrestlers, of basketball players and swimmers, and many other different sports.) So, first you must talk to your coach and decide exactly what kind of fitness you want to work for. Then the training program can begin, because you will then know what kind of training you must do.

But our job has only just begun. Let's explore more deeply the question asked earlier—what is an athlete? Then we can begin to understand just what kind of training program each athlete must work at in order to excel at his or her sport.

AN ATHLETE IS STRONG

Practically all sports require strength. Some sports require more strength than others, and some require that different muscles become strong. *Strength* is how forcefully your muscles can shorten. Muscles are attached to bones, and when muscles shorten, they move the bones that they are attached to. This is how we move. If you can make your muscles shorten very forcefully, you will move with greater force. This is important in sports. A

11

football player must be able to move with force in order to block or tackle. A basketball player must be strong also, especially under the backboard when everyone is jumping for the ball. Swimmers must be strong to get a good start off the blocks and push off the wall on turns. Wrestlers must be strong in order to break holds or perform throws. And so it goes. Practically all athletes must have great strength in one way or another, for all athletes must be able to move with force.

The best way to increase your strength is through lifting weights. By making your muscles work hard to shorten, they will become used to shortening against the weight of the barbell or dumbbell, and therefore become used to shortening in sports requiring strength. Later in this book you will see exactly how to increase the strength of your muscles by using weights.

AN ATHLETE HAS ENDURANCE

Many sports make you breathe hard and cause your heart to beat fast. When you run a great distance or work hard and fast, your muscles begin to grow tired. They need more oxygen, which is in the air we breathe. When air gets into the lungs, oxygen from the air filters into the blood, and the heart pumps the blood, along with the oxygen, to the tired muscles. The longer an athlete can work hard or run, the better his or her *endurance*. So, endurance is how well an athlete can get oxygen to the tired muscles.

The heart is important, for it is in charge of getting the oxygen to the tired muscles. You can strengthen the heart by running, bicycling, or swimming long distances. The muscles are important for endurance, too, for they have to be able to use the oxygen. Weight training can help your muscles use oxygen better: it will create more tiny capillaries to carry more blood to the tired muscles, and it will also improve the way the muscles use oxygen. Together with the heart, muscles are what gives athletes better endurance. Like strength, exercises for improving muscles' endurance are in the last section of this book.

AN ATHLETE IS FAST

The most important part of being fast is how forcefully your muscles can shorten. Being able to run with great speed means that your muscles are moving your bones very quickly. So, speed is very much like strength. Moving your body fast, as in running, requires that strength be used very quickly. This is called *power*. It is also speed. You can improve your speed by lifting weights. However, much lighter weights should be used for improving speed than for improving strength, for you must be able to move the weights very fast. We will talk about ways of improving speed and power later on.

AN ATHLETE IS AGILE

Agility is being able to change directions very quickly. For example, picture a football player carrying the foot-

13

WHAT IS AN ATHLETE?

ball. Everyone on the other team is trying to tackle him, but he dodges left and right to avoid being tackled. His ability to move quickly left and right is a good example of agility. Many athletes besides football players need to be agile. Soccer players, baseball players, wrestlers, gymnasts, and many other athletes have to be able to change directions very fast while playing their sport.

To be agile, an athlete must be fast and strong. He or she must also have good balance so that changing directions so quickly does not cause them to fall. We have already learned that speed and strength can be improved by training with weights, and so can agility, because agility is increased by becoming stronger, faster, and more powerful. Again, later in the book, we will see more clearly just what kinds of exercises are good for improving agility.

AN ATHLETE HAS GOOD BALANCE

Balance is important in many sports, whether the athlete is moving or staying in one place. *Balance* is how well you can control your body—and *muscles* control your body. Examples of balance in sports are standing on your hands in gymnastics, running with a football, jumping through the air, pole vaulting, ice skating or hockey, and many other movements. Practically all movements in sports require some kind of balance or body control. And since your muscles control your body movements, strength and power are important in improving balance.

14

We have already seen how weight training can help improve strength and power. Weight training can also help improve balance. If muscles are stronger or more powerful, they will be able to control body movements more easily as well.

AN ATHLETE IS FLEXIBLE

Two very important things happen when an athlete becomes more flexible. First, he or she can move more freely, and second, many injuries are prevented. Being flexible means that your joints, such as your shoulders, hips, and spine, are not tight. Being too fat and having muscles that are too short can sometimes cause an athlete to be inflexible. In both cases, stretching exercises are important in improving flexibility in your joints. Such exercises should be done very slowly and carefully so that the joints or muscles are not injured.

If an athlete becomes more flexible, he or she can move more freely, can do their sport skills more correctly, and therefore are better athletes. Also, being more flexible makes it harder for a joint or muscle to be injured because of the greater amount of movement that can be done.

Weight training can help to improve flexibility. By exercising muscles on opposite sides of joints, and by doing each exercise properly (through the full range of movement), tight muscles will become loose and will also become more balanced on each side of the joint.

15

Weight training can also help to lose fat, as can most types of exercise. Losing fat is a must for all athletes, for not only does being fat cause an athlete to be less flexible, but it also causes him or her to lose speed, balance, and agility. Eating too much food (especially "junk" food), and not exercising enough are what cause people to become fat. And you will rarely see an athlete who is fat.

Later on, we will see how to exercise with weights to improve flexibility, and also how an athlete should eat so that he or she does not become fat.

AN ATHLETE IS COORDINATED

Have you ever heard your coach say "Practice makes perfect"? By practicing your sport skills and having your coach tell you what you are doing right or wrong, you will become better at your sport. If you are practicing alone, you may often be doing something wrong without realizing it. That's why it is important to practice with your coach.

There is more to becoming better at sport skills than simply practicing, however. *Being coordinated* means that you are performing your sport skills the way they should be performed—that you have good control over your body movements, that you are exercising good balance, using just the right amount of strength and speed, and that you are generally fit. Being coordinated also makes it easier to learn new sport skills.

16

A physically fit person usually finds it easier to learn new sport skills because most skills require strength, speed, endurance, agility, flexibility, or balance. A good athlete has all these qualities, and also has control over his or her body movements. Once an athlete becomes fit, he or she will find that practicing sport skills with their coach is much more enjoyable, because success comes more easily.

The smart athlete knows how to become fit. This book is about becoming fit through weight training, which helps an athlete become fit and, therefore, a better athlete. Remember, an athlete becomes fit to play sports—just the opposite of those who play sports to become fit.

2: How to Become an Athlete

BECOMING GOOD at sports is not easy. Both children and grown-ups enjoy sports, and often play sports for fun and exercise, but very few people ever become really good at sports. Those who do are the athletes. It takes a lot of hard work to be one of the best in anything, and to be one of the best athletes in a sport takes a lot of hard work, also. There are three important steps in becoming a good athlete. First, you must be physically fit; second, you must eat good food in just the right amounts; and third, you must listen to your coach.

FIRST YOU MUST BE PHYSICALLY FIT

Boys and girls who want to become athletes someday must start to prepare themselves as early as possible.

18

Usually, such children do not know how to do this. In fact, they often aren't sure what sport they want to become an athlete in. Sometimes they think they do, but then change their minds as they grow older, and that's all right. The most important thing is that they prepare themselves to become athletes. That takes training in all of the types of physical fitness.

It's a bit like building a house. When you build a house, the first thing you have to do is build the foundation, the cement walls that will become the cellar. Foundations must be very strong in order to hold the house up later on. After the foundation is built, then you can build the house on top of it. That's the way it is with becoming an athlete. First you have to have a strong, solid foundation that will help you learn the skills in your sport later on—and that foundation is called physical fitness.

In the first chapter of this book, the many parts of physical fitness were discussed. It was found that physical fitness included:

1. strength
2. endurance
3. speed
4. agility
5. balance
6. flexibility
7. coordination

Also, part of physical fitness was not being fat.

(Can you remember what each of the parts of physical fitness means? If you can't, then go back to the first part of the book and read about them again. They are very important for athletes to know and understand, since they are what an athlete's foundation is built from. In the next chapter of this book, we will find out how each of the parts of physical fitness can be achieved through training with weights.)

Sometimes children know at a very early age which sport they want to become an athlete in. These boys and girls have to know which parts of physical fitness are most important for their sport, so they can become the best athlete they can possibly be. However, it is even more important for such young athletes to work on all parts of physical fitness—not just one or two of them. This is because children under twelve years old or so are still growing and need to build their foundation. Not until they have reached thirteen or fourteen years old should they concentrate only on the parts of fitness that are most important in their sport. Just as in building a new house, young athletes must first build a foundation of physical fitness. They must spend time working on all parts of physical fitness, rather than just a few of them.

PART OF BEING FIT IS EATING GOOD FOOD

Can you imagine what would happen if someone tried to build a house out of marshmallows, or if someone made your clothes out of paper? Of course they wouldn't last very long. In order to make something that is going to be strong and last a long time, you have to use good material. The same thing is true of your body. In order to build good, strong bodies that are going to last, we need good food. After all, food makes you grow, and your body is made from the food you eat.

Can you imagine what would happen to someone's body if all he or she ever ate was candy, soda, and junk food? Such a person would not be able to build a very strong body with food like that. Boys and girls who want to become athletes someday must eat good food. Otherwise, the foundation we talked about—becoming physically fit—will not be very strong.

It isn't very hard to find good food. Most mothers and fathers know what good food is. Take a look at the pictures of the different kinds of food. These show the *basic food groups*. Each day, the meals you eat should include as many of these types of food as possible. In other words, each meal should be made up of some kind of food from each of the basic food groups. Doing this will give your body all the vitamins, minerals, protein, fats, and calories it needs to become strong and healthy.

Talk about your food with your parents. Ask them to help you to become a good athlete by cooking good meals for you. Most of the time boys and girls who eat good food find that they are happier, more energetic, stronger, and not as fat. Also, parents really care about their children, and become proud of them when they learn that eating good food is one of the important steps in becoming healthy and fit.

Everyone knows that candy, soda pop, and desserts are delicious. But, of course, that does not mean that they are good for you. These types of food have a lot of sugar in them, which is why they taste so sweet. Too much sugar is very bad for anyone at any age, but it is especially bad for athletes. Athletes need good food in order to build muscle, to grow strong, and to help their bodies recover from the exercises they do.

Make a deal with your parents. Ask them to make desserts without sugar. There are many very tasty desserts that can be made without sugar, and your parents can find such recipes in cookbooks about health foods. Then ask them to buy soda pop and candy at health-food stores only. The candy and soda from health-food stores are actually good for you. They are made from good food and have very little sugar.

Having your parents do this will make it easier for you, because you will not have to give up eating candy and desserts—just give up eating too much sugar. (Remember, part of being physically fit is eating good food.) Also, when you start eating good food and less sugar, your parents may also begin to eat good foods. And parents should be healthy too.

YOU MUST LISTEN TO YOUR COACH

What is a coach? Is he or she a physical-education teacher? A former athlete? An expert at the sport he or she is coaching? Do they know how children learn skills? A truly good coach may or may not have been an athlete or a physical-education teacher. But a good coach should

(1) know a lot about the sport he or she is coaching, and (2) know how children learn skills. Part of knowing how children learn skills is knowing how children grow, how they think, and other things that make them different from adults—especially the way children grow physically and emotionally. These are the things that will someday be important in becoming a good athlete.

If you are lucky enough to have a good coach, it will be much easier for you to become a good athlete. In the first part of this book, we decided that practice doesn't always make perfect, that if you practice the wrong things, or practice with poor or incorrect form, then you weren't really becoming a better athlete. A good coach can help you practice the right things, and in the right way. A good coach knows when you are too tired to practice sport skills properly, and when you are sick or injured. A good coach can often tell if you are eating the right kinds of food. A good coach is someone that you can listen to when you are sad or when something is bothering you. All of these things are important if you are to become as good an athlete as you can be.

If, for some reason, you think your coach is not too good, or if you don't like your coach, you should do two things. First, try to be fair and decide if you are to blame, rather than the coach. Next, talk about your feelings with your parents, for they may be able to help you decide. Having a good coach whom you trust and like is very important, because then it is going to be much easier for you to learn how to become a good athlete. Your parents may decide that it would be better for you to have a new coach. Or if you and your parents decide that you have not been fair with your coach, you may want to give him or her another chance. The most important thing for you to understand is that your coach is there to help you become a better athlete. Most coaches are good, and are truly concerned about allowing you to become as good as you can be at your sport. Most of the time it is wise to give them a chance and to pay attention to what they tell you. You may be surprised at how well you like your coach, after all.

Also, good coaches know the value of physical fitness. They know which parts of fitness are most important for your sport, and how to set up a training program for each part of fitness. But not too many coaches know very much about how to train with weights. A good coach is willing to learn, so show your coach this book, for it tells how to use weight training to become fit.

3: Lifting Weights for Physical Fitness

HOW TO LIFT WEIGHTS FOR EACH PART

OF PHYSICAL FITNESS

Each part of physical fitness is different. Strength and endurance are not the same, and neither are balance, agility, speed, or flexibility. Since each part is different, the way to train for each is different. The following lists should help you in deciding how to train with weights for each part of fitness. You may notice that some things are the same, but pay special attention to the parts that are different, because the differences are what will give you good results in your training.

Training for strength (train two or three times weekly)

1. Pick exercises for those parts of the body you want to get strong.
2. Have coach or parents help you learn how to do the exercises.
3. Use a weight that you can do ten times or more.
4. Don't swing the weights up—lift them slowly ten times.
5. Rest in between each set of exercises.
6. For warming up, do the exercise with a very light weight first.

Training for endurance (train four to six times weekly)

1. Pick exercises for those parts of the body where you want to increase endurance.
2. Have your coach or parents help you learn how to do the exercises.
3. Use a weight that you can do more than twenty times.
4. Lift weights very slowly and steadily, without stopping, twenty times.
5. Go right on to the next exercise without resting.
6. Always include running, bicycling, or swimming fairly long distances with your endurance weight training.

Training for speed (train two or three times weekly)

1. Speed training almost always includes leg exercises.

2. Have coach or parents help you learn how to do leg exercises.

3. Pick a weight that you can do about fifteen times.

4. Do each leg exercise (especially squatting exercise) very fast, but be very careful not to go so fast that the weight falls from your shoulders.

5. Have parent or coach stand by you in case you fall off balance.

6. Go down only halfway in your squat position. Remember to go down slowly, but come up fast.

7. Always include short sprints and high jump-and-reach exercises with your speed weight training.

8. For warming up, do light weights slowly up and down first.

Training for agility (train two or three times weekly)

1. Remember that agility is a combination of strength and speed with balance.

2. Weight-training exercises should be done the way they are described for both strength and speed.

3. Always include running zigzag very fast in your training. Other agility exercises, such as back-and-forth sprinting and quick jumping up off the ground, should also be done.

Training for balance (train two or three times weekly)

1. Remember that balance may include strength, speed, and agility.
2. Weight-training exercises should be done the way they are described for strength, speed, and agility.
3. Always include exercises like headstands, handstands, standing on one foot, and other balance activities in your training. They will help you learn how to control your body in many other types of sport skills. Gymnastics is an especially fine sport for learning body control.

Training for flexibility (train two or three times weekly)

1. Pick exercises for those parts of the body where you want to increase your flexibility (usually shoulders and hips).
2. Be sure that each exercise you pick has a partner—that is, an exercise for the opposite side.
3. Use a weight that you can do more than ten times, and alternate your pair of exercises. In other words, do an exercise ten times and then do the partner exercise. Then repeat each of them again.
4. Be sure to do each exercise properly (through the full range of movement), and allow your muscles to be slightly stretched each time you lift the weight.

5. Never do flexibility exercises fast—go slowly and try to allow your muscles to relax when they are being stretched.

6. Always include stretching exercises such as sitting and touching your face to your knees without bending your legs, or holding a pole and bringing it over your head to your back without moving your hands. Again, do these exercises slowly, and allow your muscles to relax when they are being stretched.

So you see that there are different ways to train properly for each of the parts of physical fitness. But we also know that the most important thing for young athletes to do is to build a good foundation of physical fitness, which means that you should train for all of the parts of physical fitness, not just one or two. How can you do that? It's really quite simple. Since you should do each exercise you have chosen about three times, do one set for strength and speed, one for endurance, and the last for flexibility. Try to include as many of the other suggested exercises as possible with each weight-training workout. In so doing, you will increase your power, endurance, and speed. And because these three parts of physical fitness are the most important ones, you will also gain greater flexibility, agility, and balance.

HOW TO DO EACH EXERCISE

The following pages show pictures of each exercise that you may choose for each part of your body. The pictures

29

show the correct way to do each exercise. Next to each picture are a few words that help to explain the exercise. Study each exercise and the explanation next to it, so that you will know exactly how to perform each one. It is very important that you do your exercises in the proper way; if you don't, you may not only injure yourself, but you will not receive all of the benefit you should for each part of physical fitness. It is a good idea to have your coach or parents watch you and help you for a while, just as a safety measure, to make sure you are on the right track.

EXERCISES FOR THE ARMS

EXERCISE #1: *This exercise is called* curls. *It is used to strengthen the upper part of your arms. Two different types of curls are shown—one with a pulley and the other with a dumbbell in each hand. In both types of curls, you simply bend the elbows to lift the weight up to your chest. With dumbbells, one arm at a time is exercised, while with the pulley, both arms are exercised together.*

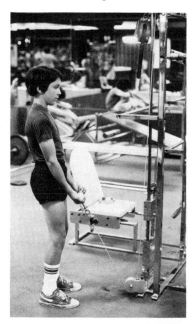 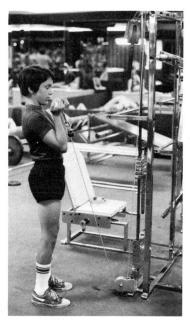

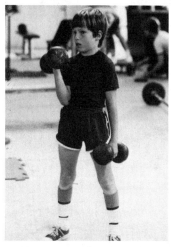

EXERCISE #2: *This exercise is called* tricep extensions, *and is done to strengthen the back part of the upper arms. Again there are two ways to perform this exercise, one with a dumbbell, and the other with a pulley. In both, the arms begin bent, and the weight is lifted by straightening the elbows.*

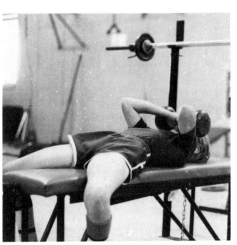
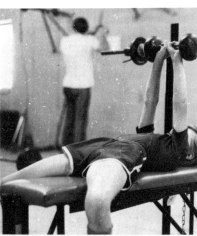

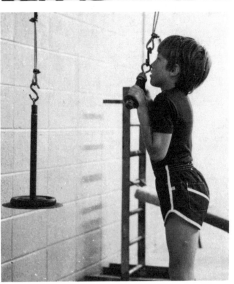
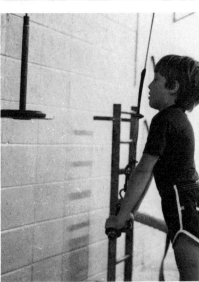

EXERCISE #3: *This exercise, called* wrist curls, *strengthens the wrists and grip. Begin with the weight far down on the fingertips, and with the muscles of the fingers and wrists, curl the weight upward.*

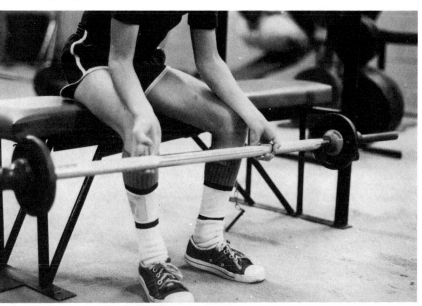

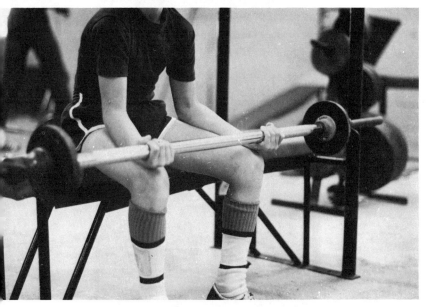

EXERCISES FOR THE SHOULDERS

EXERCISE #4: *This exercise is called* side dumbbell raises, *and is used to exercise the shoulders. Begin with the dumbbells at the side, and raise them up sideward to about shoulder height.*

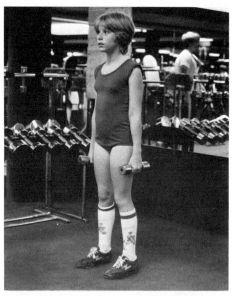

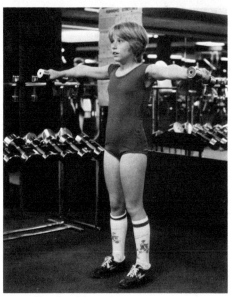

EXERCISE #5: *This exercise for the shoulders is also called* upright rows. *It can be done with pulleys or with a barbell. Begin with the weight hanging in front of you, and with a narrow grip. Pull the weight up to the chin, keeping the elbows out.*

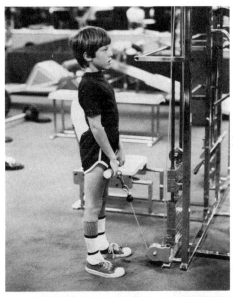

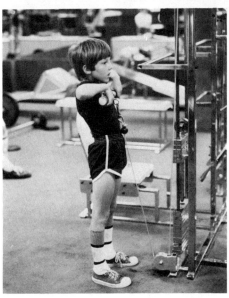

EXERCISE #6: *This exercise is for the back part of the shoulders and the upper back. It is called* inverted flys, *because the arms are moving like wings, up and down. Bending forward, raise the weights sideward until they are as high as the shoulders.*

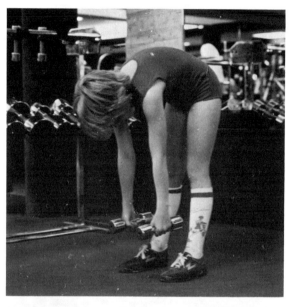

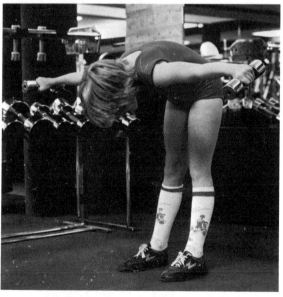

EXERCISE #7: *Here is another exercise for the back part of the shoulders and upper back. This exercise is called* bent-over rows, *because it resembles rowing a boat. Bending forward, and with the bar hanging in front of you, pull the wieght up to the chest.*

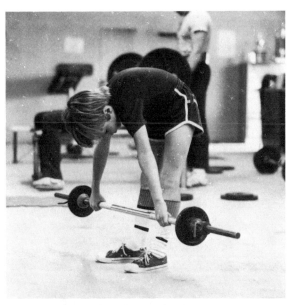

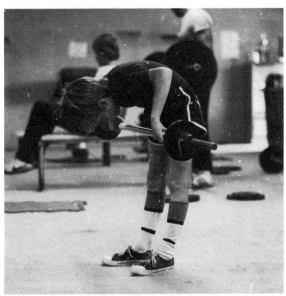

EXERCISE #8: *This exercise is called* shrugs. *It is used to strengthen the muscles on top of the shoulders near the neck, an important muscle for improving posture and shoulder stability. Simply shrug the shoulders upward toward your ears, using either dumbbells or a barbell.*

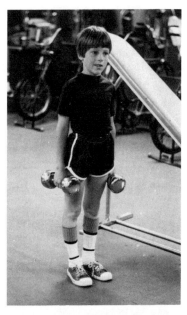

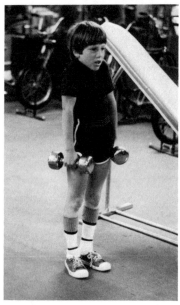

EXERCISE #9: *This exercise, called* straight-arm pulldowns, *is for the muscles in the back of the shoulders and under the arms. It is done with a pulley machine. Begin with straight arms, pulling the bar down in front of your body until the bar is at about waist level. Let the bar back up carefully so as not to jerk the shoulders, and perform the movement again for the entire set.*

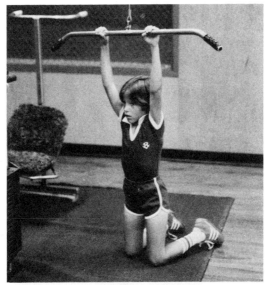

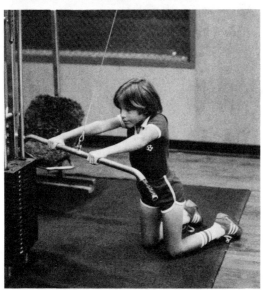

EXERCISES FOR THE UPPER BACK AND SPINE

EXERCISE #10: *This exercise is called* pulldowns. *It is for the muscles under the arms, close to the back. It must be done with pulleys. With a wide grip, and kneeling down, pull the weight to your chin.*

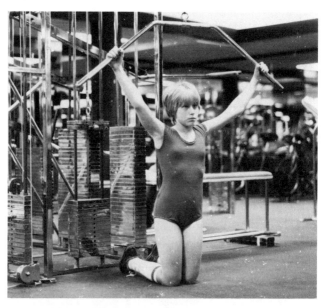

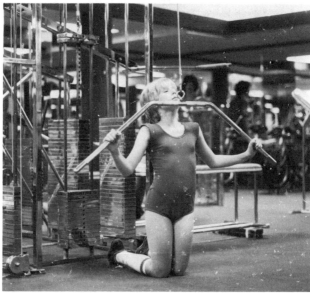

EXERCISE #11: *This exercise is called* trunk curls. *It is one of the most important exercises for young athletes, because it helps strengthen the muscles of the spine. Do this exercise slowly, and try to bend forward with the weights (either dumbbells or a barbell) by bending the spine only—not the hips. Then, after bending the spine as far as you can, slowly straighten back up.*

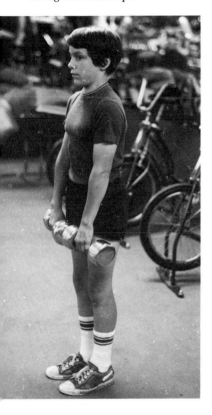 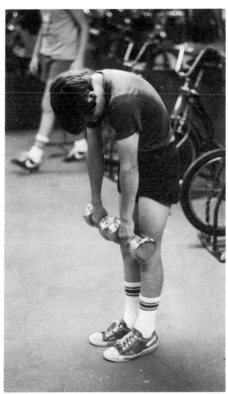

EXERCISE #12: *Here is another extremely important exercise for the spine. It is called* trunk twists, *because the spine is twisting. This exercise helps make the spine much stronger, and should be done slowly and carefully. Put weights on one end of the bar only and, with the bar across your shoulders, bend forward and point the weighted end of the bar toward the ground. Then slowly raise the weighted end so that is is pointing to the ceiling. After doing this ten times, put the weight on the other side and repeat the exercise.*

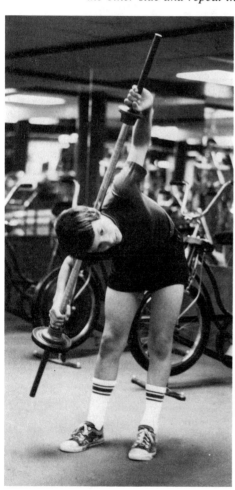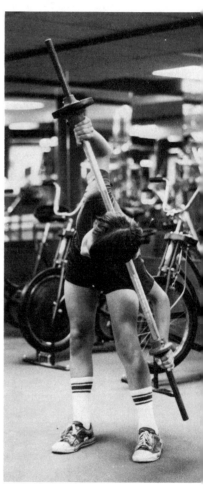

EXERCISE #13: *Some people call this exercise the* suitcase lift, *because it resembles picking up a suitcase. With your free hand behind your head (to stretch the muscles of the side), and a dumbbell in the other, bend toward the side with the dumbbell as far as possible without turning the hips. Then stand back upright. This exercise is yet another important way of strengthening the muscles of the sides and spine.*

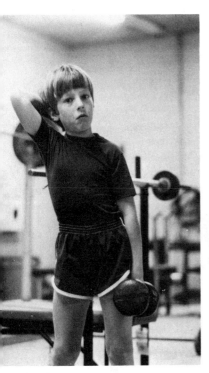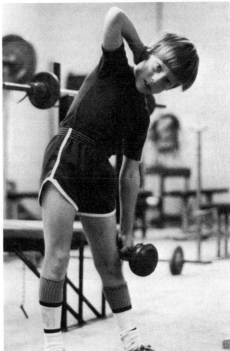

EXERCISE #14: *This is a special way of doing an old exercise that used to be called* situps. *No one should do situps all the way up, because of the pressure they cause to the lower spine. Instead, do* crunchers *to strengthen your stomach muscles. Your abdominal muscles, as they're called, really only flex the spine frontward, and do not help in a sitting-up movement. Rest your legs over a chair or bench, and, with a weight behind your head, raise your shoulders and middle back off the floor. You needn't sit up all the way. Hold the "crunched-up" position for about two or three seconds and repeat the movement ten times.*

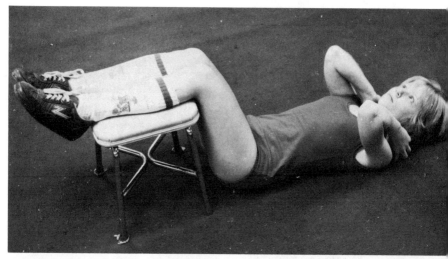

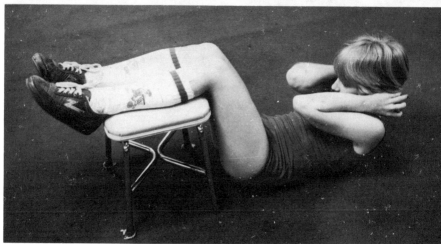

EXERCISES FOR THE CHEST

EXERCISE #15: *This exercise is called the* bench press. *It helps develop strong chest muscles, and must ALWAYS be done with a parent or coach standing by in case you miss the lift—it can be a very dangerous exercise if you try to do it alone. Even experienced weight lifters never bench-press alone. Lower the weight slowly to the middle of the chest, and press it back to arms' length. Shown below are two different ways of bench-pressing, one with a barbell, and the other with a machine. The machine is the safest way of bench-pressing because the weight can't fall on you, but the barbell is the best because it allows you to get more complete development in the chest muscles.*

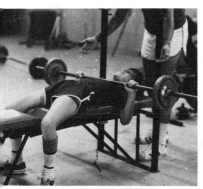
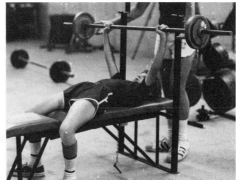
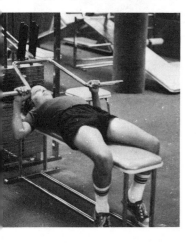
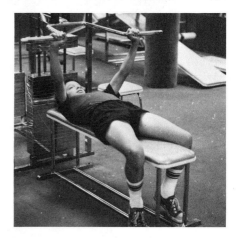

EXERCISE #16: *This is another chest exercise, called* flys *because the arms move as though you were trying to fly away. With the dumbbells in each hand, lower them to about the level of your shoulders, and raise them up to an overhead position again. This exercise can be done either with straight arms or with the elbows slightly bent.*

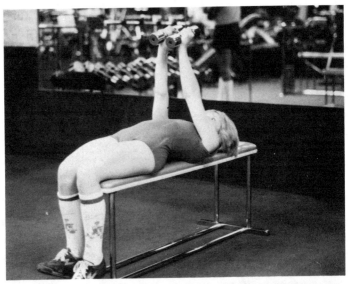

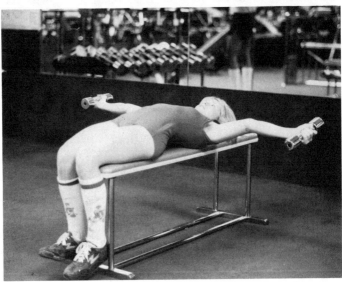

EXERCISES FOR THE HIPS AND UPPER LEGS

EXERCISE #17: *Probably the most important exercise for any athlete is the one that strengthens the hips and legs (for jumping and running). This exercise is the best of them all—*squats. *Never squat down all the way—only squat down to the height shown in the picture. Remember to keep the head and chest high, and do not slump or bend forward. Also, always have your parent or coach standing behind you to assist if you miss the lift. If you find that you cannot squat down this far without having your heels come up off the floor, simply put a block of wood under your heels.*

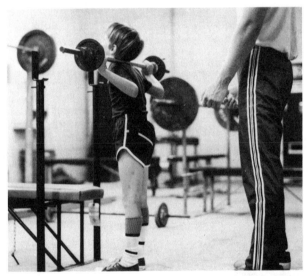

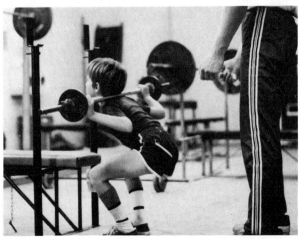

EXERCISE #18: *Here is a variation of the squat. It is done with a machine, and is called* leg presses. *While very safe, this exercise isn't as good as squats because you don't have to balance the weight as you do in the squat. However, it is still an excellent exercise for developing leg strength.*

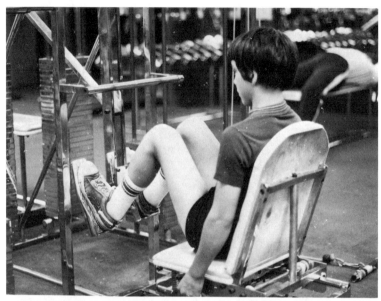

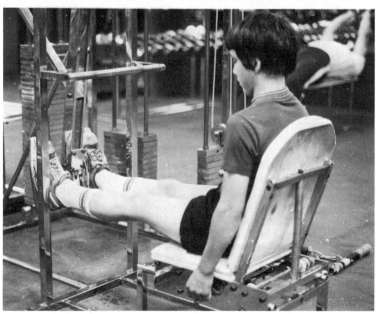

EXERCISE #19: *This exercise, done on a machine, is called* leg curls. *The muscles in back of the upper leg are strengthened with this exercise. It is one of the most important exercises for young athletes, because it helps to increase the stability of the knees. The knees are one of the most frequently injured parts of the body in sports, and must be kept as strong as possible. This is an exercise that you should do three times a week without fail.*

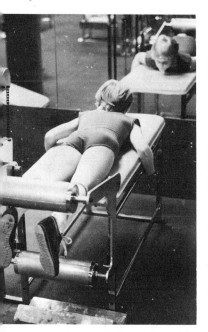
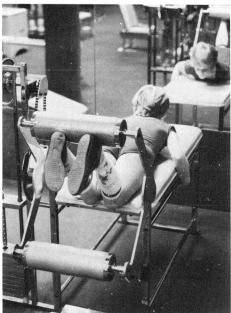

EXERCISE #20: *This exercise, called* leg extensions, *is for the muscles of the front of the leg. It helps strengthen the knees, along with leg curls. Leg extensions are dangerous for very young athletes, because of the unnatural strain they cause in the knees. Therefore, this exercise is recommended for young athletes who are over twelve years old, and only if squats (Exercise #17) cannot be done for some reason.*

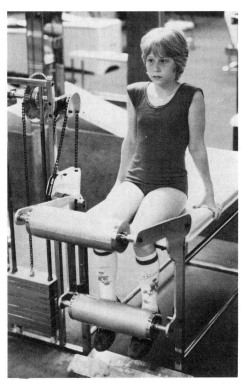 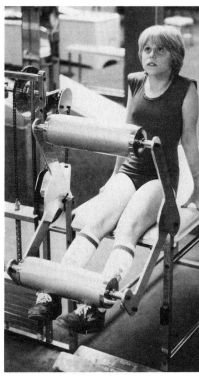

EXERCISE #21: *Here is an exercise that nearly all athletes should do. Called* high pulls, *it helps develop explosive power in the legs, back, and shoulders. Try the movement slowly at first, until you learn how to do it. From the floor, lift the weight with the legs. Then, as the bar passes the knees, begin using the back. Finally, when you're nearly straight, begin pulling the bar with the shoulders and arms until it is as high as you can pull it. When you're able to do this correctly, and with the bar staying very close to the body all the way up, then you can begin to do the exercise explosively fast.*

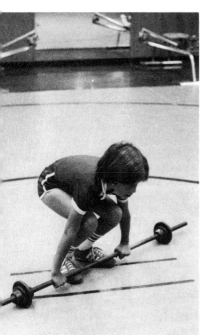 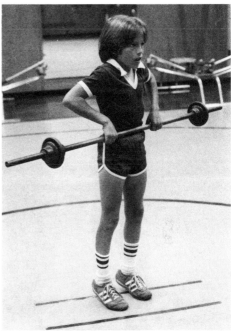

EXERCISES FOR THE LOWER LEGS

EXERCISE #22: *Most lower-leg exercises are used to strengthen the movements of the ankles. With strong muscles controlling ankle movements, you will be less likely to suffer broken, sprained, or strained ankles. These injuries are very common in sports because very few athletes ever took the time to do these important exercises. The three exercises shown here are called* toe presses *or* toe raises. *While they look different, they actually are all alike—each is done with a different piece of equipment. The top picture shows toe presses in a machine, the second shows toe raises in a calf machine, and the third shows toe raises with a barbell on the shoulders.*

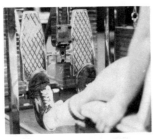 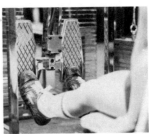

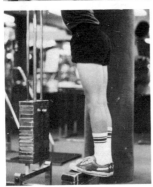 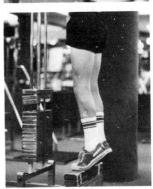

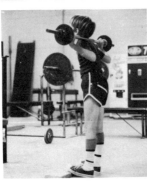 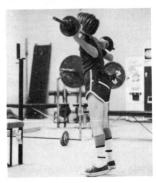

4: Some Hints for the Young Athlete

Because children are still growing, there are some important differences in the way they lift weights and exercise for physical fitness. Remember that young athletes should try to build a good foundation of all of the parts of physical fitness, rather than just a few. Once you are older—in your teens—you can begin to become more specialized, and train for your sport.

There are a few exercises that you should try to do at least once a week. They are especially for young athletes, and will help to build important muscles for later years of tough competition in your sport. They are (1) bent trunk twists, (2) trunk curls, (3) side bends, (4) leg curls, and (5) crunchers. You can find these important exercises in the exercise section of this book—the pictures show how each is done.

Doing these exercises will help you to develop a strong back and strong legs. They help to prevent injuries to the spine and knees—two parts of the body that are very often injured in sports. By doing these exercises while you are young, you will have a better chance later on of not getting hurt.

EXERCISES THAT SHOULD NOT BE DONE

Just as there are exercises that young athletes *should* do, there are also some that they should *not* do. The reasons are the same: children are still growing, they should build a good foundation of physical fitness, and they should avoid getting injured. Children should *never* try to lift extremely heavy weights. Sometimes it's fun to try to lift more than your friend, but try to remember that your muscles and bones are not yet ready for very heavy weight lifting, and in showing off, you may injure yourself. Wait until you are in your teens before you try to lift as much as you can.

Young athletes should also stay away from exercises that make them lean backward or bend their spine way back. Such exercises can injure your spine, especially down low, around the waist area. Spine injuries can be very dangerous, and can keep you from becoming an athlete. There are no pictures of such exercises in this book, because they are so dangerous. The safe thing is to

54

do only the exercises shown in this book, and in the proper way. Sometimes, a few athletes have to do flexibility exercises for their back—especially gymnasts. It is all right to do such exercises, but they should never be done with weights, and they should never be done without your coach or parents watching you.

Finally, all of your exercises should be done carefully, especially when you are stretching one of your joints. Both young and older athletes should stay away from exercises that cause the joints to stretch too much. This is important for all of the joints in your body, but especially for the shoulders, knees, and spine. Stretching joints too hard, or with too much weight, can injure them. Remember to stretch slowly and not to jerk or bounce the weights, and to stretch only a little.

SEE YOUR DOCTOR FOR A CHECKUP OFTEN

All athletes, young or old, need to be sure that their bodies are healthy, and in good repair. Your body is like a machine in many ways, and should be checked often, especially if you are playing sports. (Most grown-ups, maybe including your parents, have their car checked at a garage. Like all machines, a car needs to be kept in good repair or it will not work properly, and needs to have a mechanic check it regularly.) Your family doctor is like a mechanic in many ways, for he sees to it that your body—your "machine"—is in good working order. Without good health, you will not be able to become as good an athlete as you can be. So visit your family doctor often.

KEEPING RECORDS OF YOUR PROGRESS

All good athletes need to keep records of their training. There are some good reasons for keeping records. First of all, if you and your coach decide that something is wrong with the way you have been training, you will have a much easier time finding out the problem if you have kept records. Then, in order to make your training safer, more enjoyable, and more useful, all you will have to do is change the part of your training that was wrong.

The second reason for keeping a record of your training is so you will know when to change your workouts to match your sport schedule. During your sport's season, your weight training should continue, but with slightly more weight (a weight that allows you to do ten repetitions, but no more), and only twice a week. Before your sport's season, however, you should train with moderately heavy weights (a weight that allows you to do about fifteen repetitions), and at least three times a week. After your sport's season is over, go back to using light weights (a weight that allows you to do about twenty repetitions—but do only ten to fifteen), training three times weekly. Your coach can help you decide which other types of exercises and practice are necessary during these three periods of the year. This type of yearly schedule is called a cycle, and is used by most great athletes in practically every sport. It is very important to train according to such a cycle, because it will help you to be the best you can be when it counts—during the sport's season.

BOYS AND GIRLS BOTH BENEFIT FROM LIFTING WEIGHTS

For a long time only boys were encouraged to become athletes. Back in those days, girls had no need to lift weights, and boys didn't know how. Nowadays there are many fine athletes, boys and girls alike. Girls can become stronger, more enduring, more flexible, faster, and improve balance and coordination, just as boys can, through weight training. Girls' muscles are very much like boys' muscles, and the kind of physical-fitness activities they do should also be very similar, and that includes weight training. Weight training can help build better athletes—boys or girls.

By the time boys reach the age of thirteen or fourteen, their muscles start to grow bigger. They will grow even bigger if the right kind of weight training is used. Because they are not old enough yet, it is usually very hard for younger boys to make their muscles much bigger. With age, there are changes in boys' bodies that allow their muscles to finally begin to grow bigger. However, most girls, despite how old they are or how hard they weight-train, will never be able to get big muscles. This is because the changes that happen in boys' bodies are different from those in girls' bodies. However, girls can become stronger, faster, and more powerful. Big muscles are usually strong, but smaller muscles can also become strong with the right kind of weight training.

Boys and girls both can become better athletes through weight training, but it is wise to remember that weight training is only a part of your sport conditioning program, even though it is an important part. Remember that practice, with a good coach nearby, is important also. So are good eating habits and staying healthy.

But the most important thing for becoming a good athlete is *desire*. If you *really* want to become a good athlete, then you will do all the things that it takes to become one. Almost always, that will include weight training.

HOW TO GET STARTED IN WEIGHT TRAINING FOR FITNESS

Now that you have read this far, you are ready to begin training with weights in order to build a strong foundation in all the parts of fitness. The first step in beginning a weight-training program is to get your coach or parents to help you. Let them read this book, as they may not be familiar with how young athletes should train. Maybe they would like to train along with you. Second, you must find a good, safe place to lift weights. Most cities have good gyms or spas that have all of the necessary equipment, but smaller towns often do not. Your coach or parents may have to buy a set of weights and some basic pieces of equipment. The equipment you will need is shown in the photos of the various exercises. The most important ones are one set of adjustable dumbbells and barbell, a bench for bench presses and flys, a rack for doing squats, a pulley for the wall to do pulldowns, and a leg machine for doing leg curls. If you cannot get a leg-curl machine, try to find an "iron boot." An iron boot is a heavy shoe that straps to the foot. It is used to do leg extensions and leg curls.

You must remember that training must be done regularly, because all good athletes are very serious about their training. Good athletes rarely miss their training each day: they want to become as good as they possibly can.

5: Guidelines for Sport Conditioning

NOW THAT YOU have a good understanding of what physical fitness is, and how weight training can help you in becoming fit, you can begin to become a bit more specialized in your training. All children who want to become athletes someday should continue to train for all-around physical fitness, even after they begin to compete seriously as an athlete in their chosen sport. This means that children up to age sixteen or older should still continue to train with weights for general fitness. However, somewhere around the age of thirteen—maybe a little sooner for some, or a little later for others—some extra exercises should be added to your training. Also, the new exercises will be done in a different way, depending on the requirements of your sport. Some athletes need great strength. Others need flexibility. Still others may require speed, endurance, or power. Many athletes may need a combination of many of the parts of fitness in order to excel at their sport. So, since each one of these parts of fitness is different from the other, a good athlete will train differently for each in order to get the greatest possible benefit from training.

SOME IMPORTANT THINGS TO REMEMBER

If you want to be an athlete someday, you must do everything you can to become good at your chosen sport. If you fail to do the necessary things, it means that you are not really interested in becoming the very best athlete you can possibly be. Perhaps you are only interested in having fun or staying in shape; that's all right, but then you should not call yourself an athlete. We have already listed the things you must do in order to become the very best athlete you can be. The following pages of this book tell how to train with weights for different sports. Remember that these exercise programs are never to be done in place of general fitness exercises, but only in addition to them. You are still developing a good foundation of fitness until you are nearly through with high school, and as you now know, developing a good foundation of fitness is the most important thing a young athlete can do.

When you begin to work on developing the important skills required in your chosen sport, then, no matter what sport it is, it is time to specialize in the parts of fitness most important to your sport. As in training for general fitness, this will most often include weight training. Before you can begin such a specialized program, however, you must work with your coach in deciding exactly what parts of fitness are most important to your sport, and which parts you are weakest in. Then, you must decide exactly what muscles are most important in performing the skills of your sport, and choose the right exercises for those muscles. So, you see, it is a pretty complicated procedure, and therefore very important to get advice from a good coach.

Here are the steps you must go through in developing a weight-training program for your sport:

1. First, you must develop a solid foundation of physical fitness. The exercises listed in Chapter Three of this book are the ones that will help accomplish this.

2. After you have achieved a high level of fitness in all areas, and are near your teens, you must decide which sport you are going to try to be an athlete in. Remember that there are very few athletes who are truly great in more than one sport. This does not mean that you should not play other sports, only that you are going to concentrate on becoming as good as you can be in your favorite sport.

3. Once you have decided on a sport, you must learn all you can about it. This includes many things: knowing the rules, knowing the strategies, learning the skills, are all important. However, so is becom-

ing conditioned for your sport. You must talk with your coach and decide exactly which parts of fitness are involved in your sport, which ones are the most important, and *which ones you need the most*. Some children may already have a high level of fitness in one area, but lack fitness in another. In a case like that, the athlete should concentrate on strengthening the area of fitness he or she is the weakest in, rather than spending a lot of time on an area in which he or she is already good. You can't become fit by magic; you have to work at it, and your efforts must be very carefully planned so you can get the most out of your training.

4. Once you have decided which areas of fitness are most important to your sport, and which you need to work on most, you must decide exactly *how* you are going to exercise. All of the parts of fitness have different methods of training; for example, remember that training for strength is done differently from training for endurance. You must choose the right method. Take another look at the previous chapter to find out exactly how each part of fitness is achieved through weight training.

5. Now that you know how to exercise, you have to decide *which exercises* are the most important. Again, here is where a good coach becomes so important. Your coach can tell you exactly which muscles are the most important ones for your sport, and what exercises are the best for each muscle. You can find this out yourself, in fact, by reading

63

the previous chapters of this book. Almost all of your muscles are included in the exercises listed in Chapter Three, so you should be able to decide which exercises are best for you. You should still talk it over with your coach, just to make sure you are doing the right exercises. Remember, the best athletes are the ones who make the fewest mistakes.

6. After you have gone through all of these important steps in putting together a good weight-training program for yourself, you can begin to train. The final step is to keep good records of your training. Keeping good records will help both you and your coach in deciding whether your training is progressing as well as it should. In the back of this book there is an example of what your record book should look like. Get yourself a small notebook and copy down the things you must keep a record of, and bring your notebook to your workout every day, so you won't forget. Good records will allow you and your coach to constantly know how fit you are, whether you need new exercises, and whether you have to make changes in your present workout. In this way, you can be sure that you are getting the most out of your training.

As you grow older and into your teens, your body is constantly changing. Bones are growing longer, muscles are beginning to become stronger and bigger, and your movements and skills are getting more refined and smooth. These growth changes may make it necessary for you to constantly change your training program, because you are reacting differently to your exercises than you used to when you were younger. One of the most important things to remember as your body grows is that you are able to lift much heavier weights than before. Be very careful that you don't try to lift extremely heavy weights until you are old enough. For most children, heavy weights should not be lifted until about age fourteen or so. Until then, use a weight in each exercise you do that can easily be lifted ten or more times—never less.

SOME BASIC RULES FOR CONDITIONING IN ALL SPORTS

Nowadays, almost all athletes exercise year round for their sport, no matter what their sport is. But, depending on the time of the year, their training program may be quite different. This is necessary to ensure that they are in the best possible condition when it counts—during the competitive season, when their sport is being played. As we noted earlier, this type of yearly program is called a cycle because it is constantly changing as the year goes by. The year is usually divided into three periods: the "off-season," the "pre-season," and the "in-season." The goals of these periods are quite different. Take a look at the chart below, and you will see just how each period differs.

The important point to note about this chart is that as the in-season period draws near, more time should be

GUIDELINES FOR SPORT CONDITIONING

	Off-Season	Pre-Season	In-Season
TIME SPENT IN TRAINING	6 hours weekly	12 hours weekly	15 or more hours weekly
TIME SPENT IN ENDURANCE TRAINING	2 hours 33%	3 hours 25%	1 hour 6%
TIME SPENT IN STRENGTH TRAINING	2 hours 33%	3 hours 25%	2 hours 14%
TIME SPENT IN AGILITY AND SPEED TRAINING	1 hour 17%	3 hours 25%	3 hours 20%
TIME SPENT IN SKILLS AND STRATEGY TRAINING (ACTUAL PRACTICE)	1 hour 17%	3 hours 25%	9 hours or more 60%

spent on the skills of your sport and a smaller portion on conditioning and fitness. Since more total time is spent on conditioning and practice as the season draws near, however, even your conditioning time may increase. Always remember that the important thing about cycle training is to prepare you for the competitive season, when you will actually engage in competition in your sport: all the rest is designed to allow you to do this as well as you can. This is how to be the best athlete you can be when it counts the most—in the game!

The above chart is meant to be a guide for all young

athletes in practically all sports. As we decided earlier in this chapter, however, some athletes' needs may be different from others', and it will be up to you and your coach to plan exactly what you need the most, and to build your conditioning program accordingly.

As you grow older, your needs may also change. For example, by the time you reach sixteen years old, your skills may be very good, and your coach may decide to spend even more time developing your strength so that you can use your skills to their best advantage. Or the reverse may be true—you may be very strong but lack good skills. In that case, your coach may decide to spend more time practicing, and less time in the weight room developing strength. It all depends on your weaknesses. This is why a good coach is so important, for a good coach will always know what you need most in your training program.

Here are some basic guidelines for each of the three periods of a yearly cycle:

OFF-SEASON

This is a time when, after the in-season has ended, the athlete cuts back on his or her training time. It is a time of partial rest. However, so that it won't be too difficult to get back into shape when the next in-season period rolls around, the athlete spends most of his or her training time on conditioning, and less time on skills practice. Most athletes spend most of their off-season period in the weight room, working on the parts of fitness most important to them in their sport.

PRE-SEASON

The pre-season usually lasts for about a month or two, and is the period in which the athlete gets ready to play his or her sport. During this time, the athlete generally emphasizes refining those skills and strategies used in the game or contest. The athlete has just undergone a long, somewhat restful off-season, in which conditioning was an important factor. This conditioning achieved in the off-season will be the basis, or foundation, upon which the pre-season period training program is built. Training for strength, speed, and endurance becomes much more intense. In other words, during the pre-season, the athlete will generally lift heavier weights, run faster and longer distances, and spend many more hours in training than in the off-season, and do everything harder and faster. This will prepare the athlete for the tough in-season period.

IN-SEASON

During this period, the athlete plays his or her sport. However, since most sports are not very good for getting strong or in shape, athletes must continue to train with weights and engage in other conditioning activities. It is a very common—and serious—mistake to stop training during the in-season. All the hard work you did to become strong, fast, enduring, agile, flexible, and powerful will almost all go to waste during the in-season if you don't do something to stay in shape. If all you do during the in-season is play your sport, you will almost always

68

notice that, as the in-season passes, you will become weaker, slower, and far less explosive in your movements. This is because most sports are not hard enough to keep you highly conditioned. Although you must continue to train during the in-season, you do not have to train as hard as you did in the pre-season. Your training should include highly intense sessions once or twice weekly to keep your muscles very strong and used to explosive movement, and you should also do exercises such as running to maintain a high level of endurance. This kind of conditioning will allow you to get better at your sport, instead of worse, as the in-season progresses, and skills practice alone will not do this.

These are some of the basic guidelines the young athlete should consider when training for his or her sport. The following chapter will talk about each of the popular sports and how to weight-train for them. Thumb through the chapter and find your sport. Together with your coach, you should now have no trouble setting up a yearly cycle for yourself. Remember, everything you do is designed to make you a good athlete in the in-season. Try to leave nothing to chance. Diet, good health habits, a good coach, a sound training program, are all factors in becoming the best athlete you can possibly be.

Before going on to the next chapter, a word of caution is necessary. Remember that the exercise programs suggested in the next chapter are only guidelines. All athletes are different. They have different needs, levels of fitness, and strengths and weaknesses. So, together with your coach, decide whether the exercises suggested for each sport are the ones you need, and exactly how each is to be done. The exercises included under each sport are the ones most commonly needed by those athletes who compete in that sport. Most often your needs will be the same, but remember that they may not be—ask your coach.

6: Weight-Training and Conditioning Programs for Sports

ALL ATHLETES must work hard to be conditioned for their sport. So far in this book, ways of becoming fit have been presented, as have the definitions of each part of fitness. If you have been training properly during the years just before your teens, you are now ready to become a bit more specialized in your conditioning program. If you have never trained with weights before, but still want to become an athlete, then go back to the beginning of the book, read how to become fit, and follow the recommended fitness training program. Then, and only then, will you be ready to begin the kind of weight training the following chapter presents.

All athletes, whether they are young or in their teens, need to do certain exercises. These exercises, which are listed below, will aid in preventing injury later on. If possible, do these exercises every time you train with weights, all year long. If time is short and you can't spend more than an hour or so in the weight room, it's all right to skip them, but be sure to come back and do them the following workout. You may want to do these exercises following your regular workout.

Exercises All Young or Beginning Athletes Should Do

Exercise	Repetitions	Goal	Total Sets
CRUNCHERS	10, 10, 10	Strength	3
SIDE BENDS	10, 10, 10	Strength	3
BENT TRUNK TWISTS	10, 10, 10	Strength	3
LEG CURLS	10, 10, 10	Strength	3

FOOTBALL*

Football is one of the most popular sports in America. It is also one of the roughest, and often involves many injuries. These injuries happen mostly to the joints. Young football players especially need to have very

* The author takes a strong stand against children under the age of ten playing football in the traditional form (i.e., tackling, head-on blocking, and so forth). At this age, the skills of football should be worked on, together with a sound general fitness program—and games played only under the most controlled conditions. At puberty the child is ready to engage in the sport on a more serious level, although stringent controls and a high level of fitness remain imperative.

strong muscles to help hold joints together so that injury is less likely. Very often, a sound weight-training program can completely eliminate injuries to the joints.

Most of the time, young players (under the age of twelve) haven't decided exactly what position they want to play. So instead of training strictly for a single position, such children should train for general fitness and for general conditioning for football. After the football player is in his or her teens, he or she can then begin to train in a more specialized manner, depending upon what position he or she will play—back, lineman, special team, etc.

In the previous chapter, it was learned that athletes should divide their yearly training into three periods— off-season, pre-season, and in-season. Each one of these periods should have different goals. The goals for the off-season should be to build strength in all of the major muscles, and to increase endurance. With strength increases, the muscles will also grow in size. This is important in football, since many of the skills of football, such as tackling and blocking, depend on both size and strength. Endurance is also important since it allows the athlete to recover faster. This means that he or she will be able to play harder, and to perform skills more effectively, without fatigue hampering him or her.

Keeping these goals in mind—as well as the table in the preceding chapter, which showed how much time should be spent on each part of your conditioning program—study the workout schedule below. It is designed for off-season conditioning.

OFF-SEASON TRAINING PROGRAM FOR FOOTBALL PLAYERS UP TO JUNIOR HIGH SCHOOL

Warm-up. Follow your coach's advice. Warm-ups should include some stretching and light running exercises.

Endurance training. You should run at least two times around the football field, but not more than six times. Alternate slow, easy running with hard, fast sprints as much as you can; this will benefit your heart and lungs. For the muscles, endurance can only be increased by lifting weights. For muscle endurance you must perform each exercise for about twenty to thirty repetitions with a light weight. This is mainly important for the larger muscles of the legs, trunk, and arms.

Strength training. Weight training is the best way to make a muscle strong. Usually much heavier weights are used in strength training, but fewer repetitions are done. For strength do each exercise about eight to ten times, and always do the strength exercises before doing high repetitions for muscle endurance. Below is a typical weight-training program for young football players. Look back at Chapter Three to find out exactly how each exercise is to be done.

Exercise	Repetitions	Goal	Total Sets
BENCH PRESS	10, 10	Strength	Four
	30, 30	Endurance	

Exercise	Repetitions	Goal	Purpose
BENT ROWS	10, 10	Strength	Four
	30, 30	Endurance	
SQUATS	10, 10	Strength	Four
	30, 30	Endurance	
PULLDOWNS	10, 10, 10	Strength	Three
LATERAL RAISES	10, 10	Strength	Four
	30, 30	Endurance	
NECK BRIDGES	10, 10, 10	Strength	Three

Do the exercises listed on p. 72.

Do the exercises in order, resting no more than two minutes between sets. *Never* train by yourself. Follow your weight-training workout with some more stretching exercises.

The pre-season period's goals are to build explosive power and to become conditioned for the upcoming season. Again, as with the off-season schedule, look at the table in the preceding chapter to determine how much time should be spent in training during the pre-season.

PRE-SEASON TRAINING PROGRAM FOR FOOTBALL PLAYERS UP TO JUNIOR HIGH SCHOOL

Endurance training. Gradually begin to do only hard, fast sprints with as little rest between each sprint as you can manage. Do these about forty-five minutes each day, just before you lift weights, or right after skills practice.

75

Warm-up. Same as for the off-season.

Explosive-power training. Much heavier weights are
  normally used in explosive-power training, and
  fewer repetitions are performed. In each exercise,
  lower the weight slowly, and lift the weight as explosively as you possibly can. You must exercise
  great care, however, when doing this, because by
  lifting the weight very explosively, you may throw
  yourself off balance or perhaps injure yourself from
  the sudden movement. Lift with care, and *never*
  train alone. Do each exercise about six times in each
  set when training for explosive power (only the
  large muscles). All the other exercises should be
  done for strength rather than speed. Follow your
  weight-training workout with stretching exercises.

Exercise	Repetitions	Goal	Total Sets
SQUATS	6, 6, 6	Power	Three
CRUNCHERS	10, 10, 10	Strength	Three
TOE RAISES	10, 10, 10	Strength	Three
BENCH PRESS	6, 6, 6	Power	Three
BENT ROWS	6, 6, 6	Power	Three
TRICEP EXTENSIONS	10, 10, 10	Strength	Three
NECK BRIDGES	10, 10, 10	Strength	Three
CURLS	10, 10, 10	Strength	Three
HIGH PULLS	6, 6, 6	Power	Three

Do the exercises listed on p. 72.

The above exercises should be done three times a week (for example, on
Monday, Wednesday, and Friday).

The in-season training program's goals are to maintain the hard-won gains in explosive power and endurance that came from the pre-season program. An athlete need not train as hard or as often in the competitive season— strength and endurance can be maintained with just a little effort twice a week. Here is how it's done.

IN-SEASON TRAINING PROGRAM FOR FOOTBALL
PLAYERS UP TO JUNIOR HIGH SCHOOL

Warm-up. Same as for the off-season and pre-season.

Endurance training. Hard, fast sprints (about twenty to forty yards) should be done either after skills practice or just before weight training. Spend about thirty minutes doing sprints about three times a week.

Maintenance for strength and power. Heavy weights are used, as they were in the pre-season training program. Train twice weekly, but never within two days of your game—you need at least two days to rest before competition. Only the very important muscle groups need to be exercised during the competitive season, both for maintenance as well as for injury prevention. Stretch after each workout.

Exercise	Repetitions	Goal	Total Sets
SQUATS	6, 6, 6	Power	Three
CRUNCHERS	10, 10, 10	Strength	Three
BENCH PRESS	6, 6, 6,	Power	Three
BENT ROWS	6, 6, 6	Power	Three

77

Exercise	Repetitions	Goal	Total Sets
NECK BRIDGES	10, 10, 10	Strength	Three
HIGH PULLS	6, 6, 6	Power	Three

Do the recommended exercises listed on p. 72.

GYMNASTICS

Gymnastics for both boys and girls requires great upper-body strength. Floor exercise and vaulting require explosive leg power. Gymnastics, perhaps more than any other sport, requires great total fitness. Because gymnasts have to support the weight of their body on practically all apparatuses, and because they train on each apparatus all year long, exceptional fitness is a must. Agility, muscular endurance, power, speed, flexibility, and balance are all very important to gymnasts, regardless of the time of year—off-season, pre-season, or in-season. Therefore, gymnasts normally divide the year into two periods, rather than three. They call these two periods the "learning" period and the "performance" period. During the learning period, gymnasts concentrate on learning new tricks and combinations of tricks, both for their compulsory as well as their optional exercises. Then, once the individual skills are well learned, and just before the regular competitive season, gymnasts enter the second period. In the performance period, gymnasts spend much time on complete routines, "putting it all together" for competition.

The fitness requirements of both periods are similar for gymnasts. The only difference in the type of training with weights a gymnast will do is that during the performance period, workouts are shorter and less frequent. This is so they have plenty of time to rest before the competition and will not lose any of the strength they gained from previous workouts. Below is an example of how a gymnast will train for conditioning. The same type of program is used for both boys and girls, since the sport's requirements are similar.

YEARLY CONDITIONING PROGRAM FOR GYMNASTS

Warm-up. Follow your coach's advice. Warm-ups should include some stretching and light running exercise.

Strength training. Weight training is the best way to make a muscle strong. Usually very heavy weights are used in increasing strength, performing each exercise about eight to ten repetitions.

Muscular endurance training. In some cases, gymnasts need to be able to hold certain positions for long periods, or to do certain movements many times. This takes good endurance. Do each exercise recommended about twenty to thirty times, with slow and controlled movements, and only during the learning period.

Explosive power training. The legs are the most important part of the body in floor exercise and vaulting. Great power is necessary to perform the difficult tumbling and vaulting skills with good height. Use very heavy weights, lowering into the position slowly and carefully, and exploding through the lifting phase of the exercise. Perform about six repetitions for explosive power.

To maintain flexibility. All gymnasts need good flexibility. The exercises below are arranged in the order they should be done. By doing these exercises in this prescribed order, you will be able to stay flexible because the muscles on all sides of the joint are being conditioned. In fact, if you are inflexible, you may be surprised at how flexible these exercises will make you become!

Exercise	Repetitions	Goal	Total Sets
MILITARY PRESS	10, 10, 10	Strength	Three
PULLDOWNS	10, 10, 10	Strength	Six
	30, 30, 30	Endurance	
SQUATS	6, 6, 6	Power	Three
LEG CURLS	10, 10, 10	Strength	Three
CRUNCHERS	10, 10, 10	Strength	Six
	30, 30, 30	Endurance	
HIGH PULLS	6, 6, 6	Power	Three
STRAIGHT-ARM PULLDOWNS	10, 10, 10	Strength	Three
FRONT DUMBBELL RAISES	10, 10, 10	Strength	Three
BENCH PRESS	10, 10, 10	Strength	Three
BENT ROWS	10, 10, 10	Strength	Three

Do the recommended exercises listed on p. 72.

Always increase weights in each exercise as you become more powerful, strong, or enduring. Be sure to follow each weight-training session with a complete stretching program, and *never* train alone. Also, during the learning period, your weight-training program should be done three times weekly following your normal gymnastics workout, and only twice weekly during the competitive season.

WRESTLING

Wrestling is one of the oldest sports, dating back to the ancient Olympics. It requires great strength, explosive power, flexibility, and, above all, muscular endurance. During each of three periods, lasting three minutes each, the wrestler must repeatedly break holds, move with speed and power, execute difficult maneuvers, and display great strength in controlling his opponent. Three minutes may not sound like a long time, but by the end of the third period, the wrestler who is in condition will certainly have the advantage, and most often will win. His opponent has grown fatigued.

The wrestler's training regimen should include much endurance training, but should never neglect the important elements of power, strength, agility, and the ability to be powerful even when he is extremely fatigued. For this reason, wrestlers use a special type of training program called "circuit training," which emphasizes endurance with power. The same type of circuit is used in the off-season, pre-season, and in-season. The off-season circuit will concentrate on power and strength, the pre-season circuit on power and endurance, and the in-season circuit on maintaining power and endurance. You will notice that the pre-season circuit calls for heavier weights and less rest between exercises than does the off-season circuit. Also, the in-season circuit, while staying very fast and requiring heavy weights, is only done twice weekly instead of three or four times weekly.

YEARLY TRAINING PROGRAM FOR WRESTLERS

Warm-up. The entire circuit should be gone through once, using light weights, as a warm-up. Also, do some light stretching exercises.

Circuit training. A *circuit* is a group of exercises. The wrestler goes from one exercise to the next in a certain amount of time, and is required to complete the exercise within the time allowed. After all the exercises are done, the wrestler will go through the entire circuit a second and third time. Completing the circuit three times should be done in less than thirty minutes.

Exercises	Repetitions	Instructions
BENCH PRESS	10	Complete each exercise in thirty
BENT ROWS	10	seconds. Rest for thirty seconds
CRUNCHERS	10	and go on to the next exercise.
HIGH PULLS	10	Repeat this process until all of the
CURLS	10	exercises in the circuit have been
TRICEP		completed (about ten minutes).
EXTENSIONS	10	Repeat the entire circuit two
SQUATS	10	more times.

Exercises	Repetitions	Instructions
UPRIGHT ROWS	10	As time passes, try to increase
PULLDOWNS	10	the weight in each exercise and to
		decrease the time spent in performing the exercise and in resting. This will prepare you for the more difficult pre-season circuit training program.

Do the recommended exercises listed on p. 72.

Wrestlers should train about three times weekly during the off-season, and increase the number of times to four (every other day at least) during the pre-season. The pre-season circuit will remain the same as the off-season's, with the following exceptions:

1. Perform the first circuit doing twenty-five to thirty repetitions in each exercise. Complete the circuit in ten minutes, spending no more than one minute at each exercise.
2. Perform the second circuit doing ten repetitions with a heavier weight in each exercise. Complete the circuit in eight minutes, spending no more than forty-five seconds at each exercise.
3. Perform the final circuit doing six repetitions in each exercise with much heavier weights. Complete the circuit in six minutes, spending no more than thirty seconds at each exercise.
4. There are no rest periods between exercises or between each circuit.

5. Do all exercises explosively, being careful not to allow the weight to swing or stretch the joints.

During the in-season, follow the same circuit as used in the pre-season, but only twice weekly.

SWIMMING

In competitive swimming there are three types of races, which include short distances (sprints), middle distances, and long distances. Each of these three groups have different fitness requirements. Sprint swimming involves distances of two hundred yards and under, and requires great speed, acceleration, and power. The middle distances in swimming involve races up to about five hundred yards, and long-distance races have distances of more than five hundred yards. Middle-distance swimmers need a good mixture of both power and muscular endurance, while long-distance swimmers need to have great endurance. Because the strokes are the same (i.e., butterfly, breaststroke, freestyle, and backstroke), and involve the same muscle groups, the exercises for each group will be similar. But they will be done in a different manner, depending upon whether the swimmer needs power, endurance, or both.

Swimmers were among the first athletes ever to use weight training as part of their conditioning program. Nowadays, practically all athletes in all sports use weights for conditioning. Swimmers have developed highly scientific ways of training with weights, and often use very specialized equipment that allows them to move weights through the same kind of movements that are involved in each of the strokes. This kind of training is called "simulation" training, and is widely used by many other types of athletes as well. It is possible to get a very good training program with regular dumbbells, barbells, and other basic equipment, however; you needn't worry about getting the expensive, specialized equipment until you are near championship-level competition.

YEARLY TRAINING PROGRAM FOR SPRINT SWIMMERS

Warm-up. Do some light stretching exercises before each of your weight-training exercises. Then, do the weight-training exercises for two sets with light weights before using your normal weight.

Power training. Explosive takeoffs from the blocks, strong strokes, and explosive turns for long glides off the wall are essential in sprint races. This same explosiveness must be practiced when training with weights. Do each exercise with very heavy weights for five sets of five repetitions each. Use slow, controlled movements lowering the weight, and explosively lift the weight to the final position. Be careful to maintain balance and control of the weight, as such fast training may throw you off balance or cause injury.

Strength training. Some of your exercises are designed to give your muscles strength for stability and control, and need not be done explosively. Where strength is called for, do about ten repetitions for three sets, using slower, more deliberate movements.

Exercise	Repetitions	Goal	Purpose
PULLDOWNS	10, 10, 10	Strength	Pulling through water
LATERAL DUMB-BELL RAISES	10, 10, 10	Strength	Arm recovery and stability
CRUNCHERS	10, 10, 10	Strength	Prevent sagging in water and stability
SQUATS	5, 5, 5, 5, 5	Power	Starts and turns
STRAIGHT-ARM PULLDOWNS	5, 5, 5, 5, 5	Power	Pulling through water
BENT ROWS	5, 5, 5, 5, 5	Power	Arm recovery
BENCH PRESS	10, 10, 10	Strength	Stability and pulling through water

Do these exercises three times a week following your swimming workout. Try to increase the amount of weight as you become stronger. During the pre-season, the same exercise program should be followed, but spend very little time resting between each set and between each exercise. During the competitive season, again follow the same program, but reduce the number of sets to two for each exercise, and use heavier weights. Also, train only twice weekly instead of three times weekly.

YEARLY TRAINING PROGRAM FOR MIDDLE-DISTANCE SWIMMERS

The warm-up, power-training, and strength-training guidelines are the same for middle-distance swimmers as for sprint swimmers. Read the program on the preceding page to find out how to perform these exercises. Because middle-distance swimmers must possess good endurance as well as power and strength, they must perform their exercises slightly differently from the way sprint swimmers do.

For endurance training, lighter weight, a greater number of repetitions, and slower, more steady movements are necessary. So to get both power and endurance, middle-distance swimmers need to do each exercise both ways.

Exercise	Repetitions	Goal	Purpose
PULLDOWNS	10, 10, 10	Strength	
	30, 30, 30	Endurance	
LATERAL			
DUMBBELL	10, 10, 10	Strength	
RAISES	30, 30, 30	Endurance	The purpose
CRUNCHERS	10, 10, 10	Strength	for each
	30, 30, 30	Endurance	of these
SQUATS	5, 5, 5	Power	exercises is
	30, 30, 30	Endurance	the same as
STRAIGHT-ARM	10, 10, 10	Strength	in sprint
PULLDOWNS	30, 30 30	Endurance	swimming.
BENT ROWS	10, 10, 10	Strength	
	30, 30, 30	Endurance	

Exercise	Repetitions	Goal	Purpose
BENCH PRESS	10, 10, 10	Strength	
	30, 30, 30	Endurance	

Do the recommended exercises listed on p. 72.

Do these exercises three times a week, but alternate the days you work for strength or power and endurance. For example, train for power or strength on Monday, and for endurance on Wednesday. Then on Friday, train for strength again, and begin the next week training for endurance. It isn't necessary to do both every training day. Also, all weight-training exercises should be done after swimming practice—never before.

During the pre-season, the same exercise program should be followed, except that the exercise program should be done much more quickly, with less rest between sets, and with both strength and endurance exercises done every training day, rather than alternating days as in the off-season.

Train only twice weekly during the competitive season, and train for both strength and endurance each training day, as you did in the pre-season. Be sure to rest at least three days before the swimming meet, to give your muscles a chance to rest.

YEARLY TRAINING PROGRAM FOR LONG-DISTANCE SWIMMERS

Long-distance swimmers need great endurance in the muscles they use in their respective strokes. Long-distance swimmers do the same exercises that sprint and middle-distance swimmers do, with one important exception—all of them are done for very high repetitions (about thirty repetitions in each exercise), and, if the time schedule permits, every day. By training so frequently, great endurance can be developed. However, if you are just beginning, don't try to train every day—you must gradually work up to this kind of rigorous training schedule. Start out by training every other day, and gradually increase the number of days per week you train with weights.

As with sprint and middle-distance training, long-distance swimmers should do light stretching exercises before training, and always do their swimming workout first. Also, in the competitive season, leave at least three days to allow muscles to recover before swimming meets. Training for *muscular* endurance is just as important as training for cardiovascular (heart) endurance in long-distance events, because having a strong heart, while important, isn't going to keep the muscles from becoming fatigued. Your swimming will give you good cardiovascular endurance, but only weight training will give you the kind of muscular endurance that it will take to become a champion swimmer.

BASKETBALL

Basketball is a sport where many parts of physical fitness are essential. Great endurance for getting up and down the court, for offense and defense, is required. Explosive leg power for rebounding is a must. Great upper-body strength for those rough under-the-board scrambles for the ball is required so that you won't be easily boxed out. Great agility, for fast breaks and quick movements left and right, is also a very important part of the game for both offensive and defensive players. This kind of all-around fitness calls for a very special kind of weight-training program that will allow you to achieve all of these important parts of fitness. The truly great basketball player must be able to shoot, rebound, and play quick and agile defense under conditions of extreme fatigue— not an easy task. The kind of training program designed to achieve this ability is called "nonstop training," and in it the athlete must perform each exercise in sequence, without resting between sets. This means that each exercise is done while the heart is beating very fast—similar to what happens in a game.

Yearly Training Program for Basketball

Warm-up. Follow your coach's advice. Do light stretching exercises and easy jogging, followed by explosive agility and running drills (such as zigzag running).

Endurance training. Because the kind of endurance needed by basketball players requires explosive movements even when very tired, endurance training should be similar. Do your agility drills (zigzag running sprints described for the warm-up) back to back, with only brief rest periods. Try to gradually build up the time and speed of your sprints, and also to reduce the length of the rest periods. Spend about a half hour before your weight-training exercises doing these sprint drills.

Nonstop training. To keep the heart beating fast, go right from one exercise to the next without resting. After going through all the exercises once, repeat the sequence three more times for power exercises, and only twice more for the others. Remember, try to do these sequences without resting too much between each exercise.

Training for power. With your running drills completed, you are now ready to train for power. Explosive power is needed especially in the legs and hips for rebounding and quick offensive and defensive movements.

Training for strength. The upper-body muscles need to be strong to ensure competitiveness under the boards and body control. Strength exercises are done with slightly less weight than is used in power exercises, and are done somewhat slower and for more repetitions.

Exercise	Repetitions	Goal
SQUATS	6, 6, 6, 6	Explosive leg power for rebounding and agility
MILITARY PRESS	10, 10, 10	Arm and shoulder strength
CRUNCHERS	10, 10, 10	Stability and body control

91

Exercise	Repetitions	Goal
PULLDOWNS	10, 10, 10	Strong rebounding and ball control
HIGH PULLS	6, 6, 6, 6	Explosiveness for legs, back, and hips
BENCH PRESS	10, 10, 10	Strength under the boards
TOE RAISES	10, 10, 10	Strong calves for jumping

Do the recommended exercises listed on p. 72.

Be sure to do the recommended exercises at the beginning of this chapter as often as possible. Your pre-season training program should be identical with the off-season program described above, except that your agility drills and sprint drills must become intenser (faster, longer, and less rest between sprints). More effort must be put into the weight-training program—use heavier weights, and more explosive movements in power exercises. Also, try to complete all of the exercise sequences without resting. You should train three times weekly in both the pre-season and off-season periods. Train only twice weekly during the competitive season, using the same program as was used in the pre-season.

OTHER SPORTS

There are many, many sports that young athletes may wish to excel in besides the ones mentioned earlier in this chapter. Some of the more popular ones include:

Hockey	Ballet and Dance
Track and Field	Field Hockey
Soccer	Tennis
Baseball	Diving
Softball	Crew
Power Lifting	Skating (figure
Olympic Weight	and speed)
Lifting	Downhill Skiing
Cross-Country	Cross-Country
Running	Skiing
Boxing	Golf
Bicycling	

All of these sports require some form of conditioning if the athlete ever expects to excel in them. The basic principles of setting up a good conditioning program are the same for all sports. Go over Chapter Five with your coach, and together decide on a sound weight-training program for your sport. Remember to follow the basic principles:

1. First, develop a sound foundation of total physical fitness.
2. Be sure that the sport you've chosen is the one you wish to excel in, and get to know everything possible about your sport.
3. Identify the parts of fitness that are most important in succeeding in your sport.
4. Find out which of these parts of fitness you are weakest in.

93

5. Determine how you should exercise, and which exercises to do.

6. Train hard. Keep good records. Constantly improve on your training program as you progress toward your goal of being the best athlete you can possibly be.

Glossary

AGILITY Agility is being able to change directions very fast. To be agile, an athlete must be strong, powerful, and also have good balance.

ATHLETE An athlete is someone who participates in a sport on a very serious level. Athletes become physically fit and try to do all they can to excel at their sport.

BALANCE Balance is how well you can control your body. Whether you are running, throwing, jumping, standing on your hands, or upside down, you must be in control of your body so that you can perform your skills with accuracy and efficiency.

BARBELLS Barbells are made of iron and have a long bar with round plates at each end. Exercises are done with barbells. Barbells can weigh anywhere from twenty pounds to over one thousand pounds, depending upon the number of iron plates at the ends of the bar.

CALISTHENICS Calisthenics are a type of exercise that doesn't use barbells, dumbbells or other apparatus. Calisthenics involve using your own body as weight to perform various movements, such as pushups, situps, or jumping jacks to become more physically fit. However, calisthenics are best for flexibility, while weight training is usually better for strength, power, or local muscular endurance.

CALORIES One calorie is the amount of heat needed to raise the temperature of one gram of water one degree centigrade. But we use it to describe how much energy our bodies can get from the food we eat. All foods have calories, and it is very important that an athlete gets just the right number of calories each day. Too many will cause the athlete to get fat, while too few will cause the athlete to lose weight.

CAPILLARIES Capillaries are tiny blood vessels located very close to muscles. The muscles get their food and oxygen from the blood, and it is the capillaries that bring the blood to the muscles.

CARBOHYDRATES Carbohydrates are a type of food, usually including foods made of sugars, starches, or celluloses. The very best foods that are high in carbohydrates are vegetables, whole grains, nuts, and fruit. Sugar is also high in carbohydrates, but is not good for you in large amounts and should be avoided.

COACH A good coach is someone who knows his or sport very well. A good coach must know a lot about how young athletes learn, how they think, and how to motivate them. Having a good coach is one of the most important things a young athlete should do to become good at his or her sport.

CONDITIONING Conditioning is what athletes call their training. Not all conditioning programs involve all of the parts of physical fitness. Often they focus on developing skills that are important to the athlete's sport. However, all young athletes' conditioning programs should include a complete fitness program in order to develop a good foundation for learning a sport.

COORDINATION   Being coordinated means that all of the parts of the body are working together efficiently. It means that you are performing with skill as a result of good practice and physical fitness. It takes just the right amount of practice and fitness to become coordinated in any sport.

CYCLE   A cycle lasts one year. Most cycles of training are divided into three time periods: (1) off-season period, when weak skills and fitness are worked on, (2) pre-season period, when slightly heavier training prepares the athlete for the coming season, and (3) the in-season period, when the athlete is playing his or her sport, but is also lifting weights and engaged in other training to maintain good fitness and improve weak skills. Almost all good athletes train year-round for their sport and use cyclic training.

DUMBBELLS   Dumbbells are like barbells, only smaller. The bar is about 12–15 inches long, and the iron plates at each end of the bar are fairly small. Dumbbells are held in one hand, while barbells require the use of both hands.

ENDURANCE   Endurance is how well oxygen can be supplied to tired muscles. The heart is important, for it takes care of getting the blood to the muscles. But the muscles themselves must be able to use the oxygen efficiently. Training improves both the heart's ability to transport blood, and the muscles' ability to use oxygen. A good measure of endurance is how quickly you can recover from fatigue and how long you can run.

FAT   Like carbohydrates, fat is a type of food. Fat provides us with energy, although carbohydrates are better since it is very difficult to use fat in our bodies. Most people eat far too much fat in their meals. Less than one fourth of an athlete's diet should be fat. Fat comes from animals (meat), nuts, vegetables, and dairy products.

FITNESS Being physically fit means that all of the parts of fitness are developed as much as possible. The parts of physical fitness include strength and power, speed, balance, flexibility, agility, endurance, and coordination. Young athletes need to be physically fit, while grown athletes generally concentrate more on the parts of fitness that are important in their sport, but work on general fitness as well.

FLEXIBILITY Being flexible means that your joints can move easily without tight muscles limiting their movement. Athletes need to be flexible to avoid injuries and to be better at their sport skills. Proper stretching exercises and weight training helps to improve flexibility.

FOOD GROUPS There are four basic food groups, including: (1) meats, fish, and fowl, (2) vegetables and fruits, (3) milk and dairy products, and (4) breads and cereals. Each group provides very important vitamins, minerals, and protein, so it is important that each meal contain food from each of these groups. It is especially important for athletes, since they want their bodies to work as efficiently as possible.

FOUNDATION For all young athletes, building a strong foundation of physical fitness is very important. All of the parts of fitness should be improved at a young age, so that participation in sports will be more enjoyable and less bothered by injuries, and you will be better able to learn the skills of your sport.

HEART The heart is a muscle. It pumps blood around the body, carrying with it oxygen and food and energy for muscles. Building a strong heart is important for most athletes, because most sports require at least some endurance. A strong heart, together with trained muscles, is important in increasing an athlete's level of endurance.

JUNK FOOD   Junk food is any type of food that has too much sugar in it or is not nutritious. It's called junk because it's not good for you and it contributes to becoming fat and unhealthy. Examples of junk food are not hard to list in most parts of the United States, for they are very popular because they taste so good. Good taste does not make them good for you, however. Athletes should stay away from junk food as much as possible, in order to build a strong foundation of fitness.

MINERALS   Minerals are another type of nutrient and are found in most foods. They perform many useful and necessary tasks in our bodies. They produce energy, help build muscle, help repair our bodies, and help control many body functions. Eating foods from all of the basic food groups each meal will give your body all the minerals it needs.

MUSCLE   Muscles are what cause us to move. When muscles shorten, they pull at bones and the joints bend. Strong muscles help to move us more easily than weak muscles. Athletes need strong muscles because that's what sports are all about—movement! Athletes also need muscles that have endurance, because often movements in sports have to be done over and over without tiring. Most of the exercises you do, especially weight training, are designed to give you stronger and more enduring muscles.

NUTRITION   Good nutrition means that all of the types of food important to building strong bodies are included in each of your meals. A nutritious meal will consist of all of the four basic food groups. Each meal, then, will contain carbohydrates, fats, protein, vitamins and minerals in just the right amounts.

OSGOOD/SCHLATTER'S DISEASE   Athletes between the ages of about ten and fourteen often begin to have sore knees. A large, painful bump appears just below the knee. This is very often Osgood/Schlatter's Disease. It can often be prevented. Training with weights for a couple of years before the age of ten, including especially leg curls for the back of the leg, helps to prevent the bump on the knee from appearing. This is very important for athletes, since having sore knees can keep you from becoming good at your sport. Getting a regular checkup by your doctor is also a good idea, for he can tell you other ways of preventing Osgood/Schlatter's Disease.

POWER   Power is strength with speed. Being able to move explosively fast or jump very high or far are examples of power. Training with weights helps to increase power better than any other type of exercise.

PROTEIN   Like fats and carbohydrates, protein is one of the three types of food. It is important in building muscles. About one fourth of your food each day should be protein. The very best source of protein is eggs. Milk, meat, and fish are very good protein foods also.

SPEED   Speed is how fast you can move. Running, spinning, twisting, and arm or leg movements are examples of movements in sports that require speed. Since muscles are what moves our bodies fast, without strong, powerful muscles, an athlete is not going to be as fast as he or she can be. And, isn't part of being an athlete to be as good as you can be?

STRENGTH   Strength is how forcefully your muscles can shorten. The more force your muscles can produce, the stronger you are. Training with weights is by far the best way to become strong. All sports require strong muscles, and many of the other parts of fitness depend on how strong your muscles are.

VITAMINS   Vitamins are one of the nutrients our bodies need to grow and to stay fit and healthy. Vitamins do many things in our bodies, but the most important job is to help us make energy so that our muscles can work, grow, and recover from heavy work or exercise. All the vitamins you need are found among the four basic food groups. If each meal contains at least one type of food from each of the four food groups, chances are that you will get all of the vitamins your body needs.

WEIGHT LIFTING   Weight lifting is a sport, just like basketball, gymnastics, track and field, or any other. Do not confuse weight lifting with weight training! Training with weights is not the same as weight lifting. All athletes should train with weights, and athletes who do weight lifting also use a weight training program to get in shape.

Appendix One

Some Calisthentics That
Can Be Done When Weights
Are Not Available—
or for Warming Up

NECK BRIDGES

Here is an exercise that is extremely important for football players and wrestlers. Many other sports also require good strength in the muscles of the neck. It is called neck bridges *because your body forms a bridge. The weight of your body is resting partly on the head, which is supported by the neck muscles. Be extremely careful doing this exercise—have your coach or parent watch you so that yo do not go back too far on your head or too far to the side. Slowly and carefully, raise your body up and down by pressing the back of your head into the mat. Do not do quick, jerky movements in this position.*

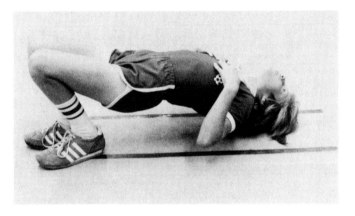

PUSHUPS

Pushups can be done two different ways. Both are for the chest muscles mostly, but also are good for the shoulders and arms. One way is to do them on the floor, being certain that the body remains rigid at all times—don't sag in the midsection. The other way is to do them between two chairs or benches, allowing your body to go a little lower than it could on the floor. This is a more difficult kind of pushup than floor pushups. It also is mainly for the chest. If you can do more than twenty pushups, then have your coach or parent apply a little pressure on your shoulders when you're pushing up—this will make the exercise more difficult—and more effective.

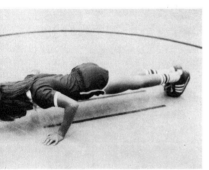 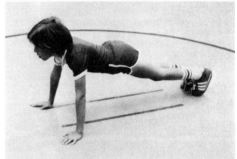

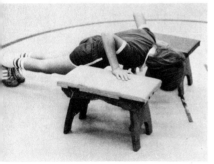 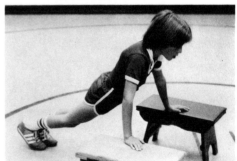

DIPS

This exercise is called dips *because you must dip your body up and down between two chairs. It is an excellent exercise for the front part of the shoulders as well as for the arms. If you can perform this exercise more than twenty times, then it would be a good idea to have your parent or coach apply a little pressure downward on your shoulders while you're coming up to make it a bit more difficult. Also, you may want to try a really hard method of doing dips—in between a set of parallel bars with your body hanging straight down.*

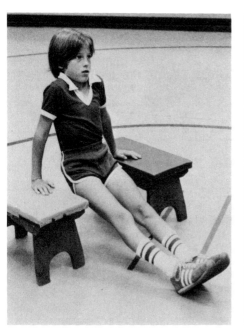 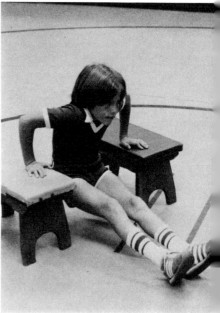

MODIFIED PULLUPS

Everyone knows what pullups are. The athlete hangs from a bar and pulls the chin over the bar using the arms. But most young athletes can't do these difficult pullups for enough repetitions to produce as much strength as possible. So a "modified" pullup should be done instead. You will notice that the young athlete in the picture is still pulling his body up so that his chin is above the level of the bar, but his body is at an angle, with his feet resting on a bench. This makes the exercise a bit easier to perform, and allows the athlete to perform the appropriate number of repetitions for greater strength.

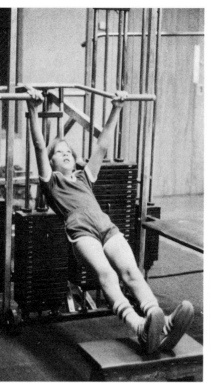
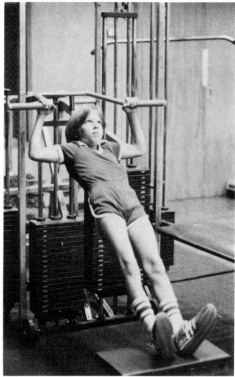

CRUNCHERS

These exercises, actually modified situps, are called crunchers *because you must "crunch" your body together with your abdominal muscles. One kind is done with the legs over a chair or bench, and the athlete tries to bring his/her ribs closer to the hips using the stomach muscles. The other, called* reverse crunchers, *requires that the athlete bring the hips closer to the ribs. This is accomplished by drawing the knees up until they touch the forehead. All athletes need a strong midsection because it makes it easier to hold the upper body or lower body stable while performing sport skills.*

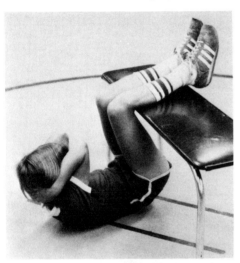 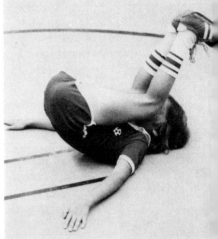

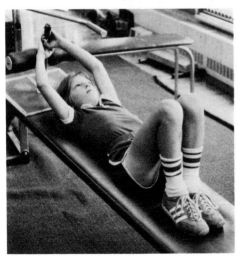 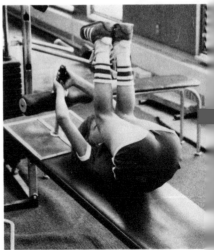

Appendix Two

*Some Stretching
Exercises to Be Done for
Flexibility Before and
After Workouts*

SEATED SHOULDER STRETCH

An excellent way to loosen up your shoulders is to perform the shoulder-stretch exercise. Leaving the feet in place, and your hands in place behind you, slide your seat closer to the feet. This will cause the shoulders to get stretched. You must do this exercise slowly, and try to relax the tight muscles rather than stiffening them up when pressure is applied. Spend about three or four minutes in this stretched position.

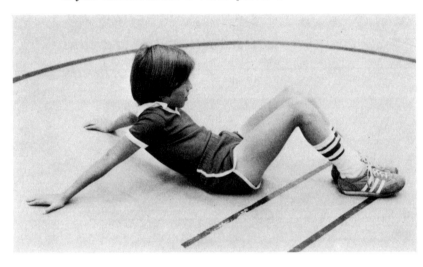

SHOULDER STRETCH WITH POLE

The shoulders are required to be flexible in almost all sports, not only to prevent injury, but also so that the athlete can get into good positions for various sport skills. Here are two ways to stretch the shoulders using a broomstick. One way, called dislocates, *involves holding the pole in both hands and bringing the pole over the head to the back of the body without moving the hands or bending the elbows. As you become more flexible, you will find that you can accomplish this with your hands even closer than the boy in the picture has his. The second way to use a pole for shoulder flexibility is to hold the pole behind the back with one hand over the shoulder, and the opposite hand under, as shown. By tugging gently downward with the bottom hand, the top shoulder is stretched, and while tugging gently upward with the top hand, the opposite shoulder is stretched. With both methods care must be taken to relax the tight muscles and not to perform the exercise in a jerky fashion—slow, easy stretching is always better than bouncing or jerking.*

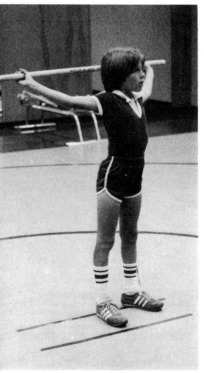
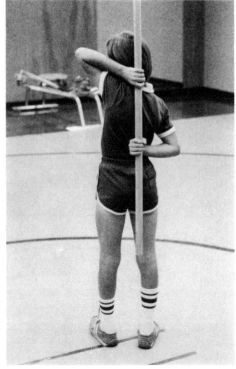

TRUNK TWISTS

Here is an exercise that helps loosen up the muscles of the spine and shoulders. Hold a broom handle on your shoulders and twist from side to side, slowly at first, then a little faster. Do not go so fast, however, that you put too much strain on the spine at either end of the movement—moderate speed is best.

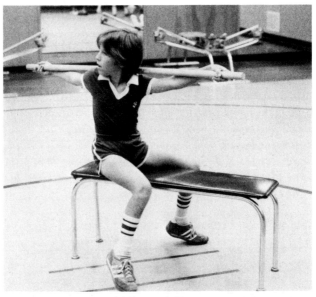

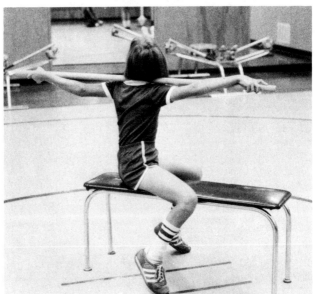

HAMSTRING STRETCH

The hamstring muscles are located in the back of the upper leg, and are the most common muscles to become tight. Injuries to this group of muscles occur often in sports, so it is very important to do whatever you can to keep them loose. Two common ways of stretching these muscles are shown here. One involves standing up and pulling your chest closer to your knees by tugging gently at the lower legs. The other is done the same way, but in a seated position and with the legs spread apart. This second way is also a good way to stretch the muscles in the groin area, between your legs—the farther apart your legs are, the more the stretch is to the groin muscles. Both types of hamstring-stretching exercises must be done slowly, without bouncing. Also, try to relax the tight muscles, and stay in this relaxed, stretched position for about two or three minutes. Remember, you must concentrate on relaxing the tight muscles—if they become tense, then stop for a while.

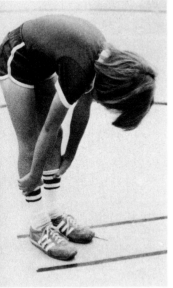 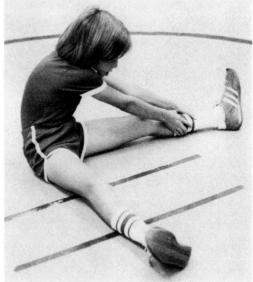

THIGH STRETCH

The thigh muscles are in the front part of your upper legs. If these muscles are too tight, an athlete can more easily get injured. To stretch these muscles out and make them looser, sit on your heels and lean backward gently, supporting your weight with your hands. Gradually lean farther back, relaxing the tight muscles as you do so. Stay in this relaxed, stretched position for about three or four minutes.

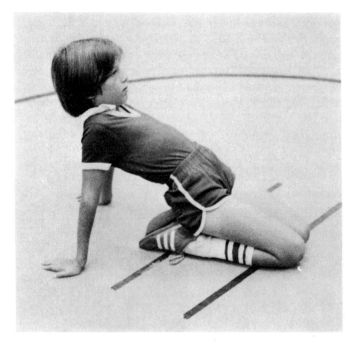

ANKLE STRETCH

Ankle inflexibility is a common cause of injury among athletes. You can stretch the ankles by leaning toward a wall and trying to touch your knees to the ground in front of you without allowing the heels to come off the floor. Again, do this exercise slowly and try to relax the tight muscles. Stay in the stretched, relaxed position for about two or three minutes.

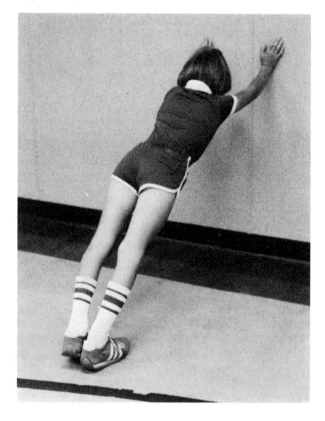

Appendix Three

*An Example of an Athlete's
Training Record*

WEEKLY LOG OF WORKOUTS

DATE _____ SYSTEM _____
(pre-, in-, off-season)

Exercises (in sequence)	1st Day			2nd Day			3rd Day		
	sets	reps	wt.	sets	reps	wt.	sets	reps	wt.

Comments (how you feel, progress, problems, suggested remedies, and other factors affecting your training):

Routine changes made this week:

ABOUT THE AUTHOR

Dr. Frederick C. Hatfield is the coordinator of the weight-training and conditioning programs at the University of Wisconsin/Madison. He received his Ph.D. degree in physical education at Temple University in Philadelphia. For the past eight years Dr. Hatfield has been ranked among the top five Olympic weight lifters in his body-weight division in the United States. He holds a world record and the American record in his body-weight division in the sport of power lifting. During his undergraduate career, Dr. Hatfield was a gymnast; he competed in three NCAA championships and won the New England championships on the horizontal bar. To his credit are more than one hundred awards in the sports of track and field, gymnastics, Olympic weight lifting, power lifting, and body building. Dr. Hatfield has written many articles and books in the field of weight training and conditioning.